RECENT ADVANCES IN HEMATOLOGY RESEARCH

THROMBOCYTOPENIA

EPIDEMIOLOGY, POTENTIAL COMPLICATIONS AND EMERGING TREATMENTS

RECENT ADVANCES IN HEMATOLOGY RESEARCH

Additional books in this series can be found on Nova's website under the Series tab.

Additional e-books in this series can be found on Nova's website under the e-book tab.

RECENT ADVANCES IN HEMATOLOGY RESEARCH

THROMBOCYTOPENIA

EPIDEMIOLOGY, POTENTIAL COMPLICATIONS AND EMERGING TREATMENTS

MCKENZIE G. BELL
EDITOR

New York

For permission to use material from this book please contact us:
Telephone 631-231-7269; Fax 631-231-8175
Web Site: http://www.novapublishers.com

Library of Congress Cataloging-in-Publication Data

ISBN: 978-1-63321-713-3

Library of Congress Control Number: 2014947417

Published by Nova Science Publishers, Inc. † New York

Contents

Preface

Decreased platelet counts can be due to a number of disease processes causing decreased platelet production, increased platelet destruction, or can be medication-induced. Health care providers have to differentiate inherited thrombocytopenias, primary immune thrombocytopenias (ITP), secondary immune thrombocytopenias, myelodysplastic syndromes with thrombocytopenia, bone marrow failure syndromes and non-immune thrombocytopenias. ITP is the most common cause of isolated thrombocytopenia. This book focuses on discussing ITP in adults; new treatment for ITP; thrombocytopenia during pregnancy; the different diagnosis of thrombocytopenia; heparin-induced thrombocytopenia; and thrombocytopenia in dengue.

Chapter 1 - Immune thrombocytopenic purpura (ITP) in adults is a common platelet related condition seen by clinicians in all disciplines. In this chapter, the authors will discuss the following topics related to this disease: epidemiology, the definition of the problem, clinical presentation, diagnosis including laboratory evaluation and the differential diagnosis, the underlying pathophysiology as the authors understand it, treatment options including first and second line therapies and finally how to manage ITP during special circumstances such as in the surgical patient and during pregnancy. At the conclusion of reading this chapter, the clinician should have a greater understanding of this disease.

Chapter 2 - Thrombocytopenia in the hospital setting is a common platelet related condition seen by clinicians in all disciplines. It may be the result of something acquired during that hospitalization or in the recent past or in some circumstances even after a recent hospitalization, or it can be result of a congenitally acquired disorder. In this chapter, the authors will discuss the following topics related to this disease: how infections and medications impact this disorder; the impact of some common medical conditions that predate a hospitalization and how these diseases may impact upon a patient with thrombocytopenia; the causes of severe thrombocytopenia as defined as a platelet count of less than $10,000/mm^3$ and thrombocytopenia as it relates to pregnancy. The authors will discuss various aspects of these issues including the epidemiology, the definition of the problem, clinical presentation, diagnosis including laboratory evaluation and the differential diagnosis, the underlying pathophysiology as the authors understand I and, treatment options. At the conclusion of reading this chapter, the clinician should have a greater understanding of this spectrum of this problem.

Chapter 3 - Immune thrombocytopenic purpura (ITP) is an autoimmune disorder characterized by an immune response against the host's own platelets. The goal of treatment is to keep the platelet count above 30 x10^9/L to prevent major internal organ bleeding. The initial therapy involves high dose steroids and or intravenous immunoglobulin IVIG. If unsuccessful, other immunosuppressant agents or biologic agents are used. Splenectomy also has been used with variable response. All of these therapies have considerable toxicity.

In the past the authors have identified a subset of patients who were refractory to treatment. These ITP patients had positive ANA's and were vitamin D deficient. Clinically they had SLE and Sjögren's syndrome overlap syndrome. Their response to high dose vitamin D replacement and hydroxychloroquine was dramatic. Their platelet counts normalized, but upon discontinuation of high dose vitamin D, platelet counts plummeted. With reinstitution of vitamin D, platelet counts were again restored. No untoward side effects were observed.

Recent research has shown that vitamin D deficiency is associated with increased cardiovascular risk, osteoporosis, cancer, diabetes type I in children, and autoimmune diseases such as multiple sclerosis and Crohn's disease. Previously the authors found an association between vitamin D deficiency and immune thrombocytopenia. There may also be synergism between vitamin D supplementation and hydroxychloroquine. Vitamin D has long been thought to play an immunomodulatory role. Specifically, 1,25(OH)2D3 seems to have two important functions: down regulation of over proliferative CD4+ cells and up regulation of T regulatory cells.

Chapter 4 - Platelet counts falls progressively in pregnancy, although usually remains within the lower normal limits. In the third trimester, platelet count can fall to 100x109/l 150x109/l, in the absence of pathological process. Hence, thrombocytopenia is a common finding in pregnancy. Most cases are mild and have no significance for mother or fetus but, in some instances, where thrombocytopenia is part of a complex clinical disorder, there can be profound and even life-threatening consequences for both mother and baby. The commonest cause includes Gestational thrombocytopenia and accounts for 75% of cases of thrombocytopenia in pregnancy and has an incidence upto 8% of all pregnancies. It is a benign condition usually occurs incidentally later in pregnancy and there is no bleeding risk to mother or fetus. Many of the features are similar to mild immune thrombocytopenia (ITP) and it can be difficult to distinguish between the two disorders. There are no specific diagnostic tests for either and both conditions are diagnoses of exclusion.

ITP is usually a chronic condition, often occurring among young women. The incidence is estimated at 0.1-1/1000 pregnancies, accounting for approximately 3% of cases of thrombocytopenia in pregnancy. It is a diagnosis of exclusion, although in approximately two-thirds of cases the diagnosis is already established before pregnancy, allowing the opportunity for pre-pregnancy counselling.

Thrombocytopenia in ITP is predominantly caused by antibodies that are specific to platelet surface glycoproteins - which bind to the platelets in the maternal circulation, resulting in immune-mediated platelet destruction. Recent research suggests there is also suppression of platelet production. The antibodies can cross the placenta and cause fetal thrombocytopenia. The aim of management is to maintain an adequate platelet count that will minimise the risk of bleeding during pregnancy, delivery and postpartum period. Platelet counts should be closely monitored throughout pregnancy.

The majority of women will not require treatment in the antenatal period, treatment is more often required to increase the count before delivery. Prednisolone is the usual first-line choice but some women may need intravenous immunoglobulin (IVIg) to increase counts rapidly. Rarely, Anti-D immunoglobulin appears be useful for women who are rhesus positive.Both these options are useful when a rapid increase in platelet count is required.

The other rarer causes of thrombocytopenia include Thrombotic thrombocytopenic purpura, Haemolytic Uremic Syndrome, Hereditary Thrombocytopenia, Pseudothrombocytopenia, Viral infection, drugs and lekemia and lymphoma.

Chapter 5 - Decreased platelet counts can be due to a number of disease processes causing decreased platelet production, increased platelet destruction, or can be medication-induced. The authors have to differentiate inherited thrombocytopenias, primary immune thrombocytopenias (ITP), secondary immune thrombocytopenias, myelodysplastic syndromes with thrombocytopenia, bone marrow failure syndromes and non-immune thrombocytopenias. ITP is the most common cause of isolated thrombocytopenia.

There are three diagnostic cornerstones for diagnosing ITP – patient history, physical examination, and peripheral blood smear confirming thrombocytopenia to exclude pseudothrombocytopenia. Other tests recommended to establish ITP diagnosis are direct antiglobulin test and tests for *Helicobacter pylori*, HIV and hepatitis C.

Chapter 6 - Heparin induced thrombocytopenia (HIT) is a highly prothrombotic disorder mediated by platelet activating immunogloubulin G antibodies that bind to conformational epitopes on platelet factor 4 (PF4) when it is complexed with heparin. HIT occurs in 0.2% to 5% of adults treated with heparin. The risk is higher with the use of unfractionated heparin, longer duration of therapy, older women and surgical patients. HIT can present with isolated thrombocytopenia, thrombosis or other unusual manifestations. Typically, platelet count drops by $\geq$ 50% from baseline, beginning 5 to 10 days after the initiation of heparin therapy. However "rapid-onset" HIT and "delayed-onset" HIT can present diagnostic challenge. Approximately half of the untreated cases of isolated thrombocytopenia can develop thromboembolic events, predominantly venous thromboembolism. HIT is paradoxically under-recognized and over-diagnosed. As such, the current diagnostic algorithm utilizes both pre-test clinical probability and the results of laboratory assays. The widely utilized risk assessment system (4Ts score) provides an estimate of the pre-test probability of HIT by assigning scores based on the degree of thrombocytopenia, the timing of the drop in the platelet count, the presence of a thrombosis and the exclusion of other causes of thrombocytopenia. Laboratory diagnosis relies on the determination of the presence of circulating anti-PF4/heparin antibodies (immunologic assays) or the ability of such antibodies to cause platelet activation (functional assays). Enzyme linked immunosorbent assay has excellent sensitivity but suffers from poor specificity because of the detection of non-pathogenic anti-PF4/heparin antibodies. Functional assays such as serotonin release assay have significantly higher specificity but are not widely available. Treatment of HIT includes immediate withdrawal of all heparin products, initiation of a non-heparin anticoagulant (frequently argatroban) and transition to warfarin once the platelet count has normalized. Anticoagulation is maintained for at least 4 to 6 weeks in cases with isolated thrombocytopenia, and at least 3 months with thrombosis.

Subcutaneous fondaparinux has emerged as an alternative agent for the management of HIT. Multiple small case series have demonstrated comparable efficacy to argatroban and lepirudin, and excellent safety profile. Additionally, its fixed weight-based dosing and subcutaneous route prevents the need for frequent monitoring and allows easier transition to warfarin. Consequently, in the absence of kidney dysfunction, some experts utilize it as the therapy of choice in HIT. Conversely, there are documented cases of fondaparinux-associated

HIT as well as worsening of HIT with the use of therapeutic fondaparinux. Although fondaparinux offers several advantages over alternate therapeutic options, such instances require carefulness during its use for the management of HIT.

Chapter 7 - Dengue is an important tropical infection caused by dengue mosquito vector. Annually, thousands cases of dengue can be seen in tropical zone. This infection classically manifests as an acute febrile illness with thrombocytopenia. Thrombocytopenia in dengue can be problematic and lead to fatality. Several complications of dengue thrombocytopenia can be seen in tropical medicine. In this brief article, the authors will review and discusses on the complication of dengue thrombocytopenia and its treatment.

In: Thrombocytopenia
Editor: Mckenzie G. Bell

ISBN: 978-1-63321-713-3

Chapter 1

Immune Thrombocytopenic Purpura (ITP) in Adults

Alida Podrumar, MD[1,*], Gita Lisker, MD[2,†], Debra A. Ferman, MD[1,‡] and Alan S. Multz, MD[1,§]
[1]Nassau University Medical Center, East Meadow, NY, US
[2]North Shore Long Island Jewish Health System, NY, US

Abstract

Immune thrombocytopenic purpura (ITP) in adults is a common platelet related condition seen by clinicians in all disciplines. In this chapter, we will discuss the following topics related to this disease: epidemiology, the definition of the problem, clinical presentation, diagnosis including laboratory evaluation and the differential diagnosis, the underlying pathophysiology as we understand it, treatment options including first and second line therapies and finally how to manage ITP during special circumstances such as in the surgical patient and during pregnancy. At the conclusion of reading this chapter, the clinician should have a greater understanding of this disease.

Keywords: Immune thrombocytopenic purpura, thrombocytopenia

* Alida Podrumar, MD: Nassau University Medical Center, 2201 Hempstead Turnpike, East Meadow, NY 11554. (P): 516-572-6501, (F): 516-572-5609, e-mail: apodruma@numc.edu, alida70@hotmail.com.

† Gita Lisker, MD: North Shore Long Island Jewish Health System, 410 Lakeville Road, Suite 107, New Hyde Park, NY 11040. (P) 516-465-5433, e-mail: Glisker2@nshs.edu, gitalisker@yahoo.com.

‡ Debra A. Ferman, MD: Nassau University Medical Center, 2201 Hempstead Turnpike, East Meadow, NY 11554. (P): 516-572-6501, (F): 516-572-5609, e-mail: fermantor@optonline.net.

§ Corresponding author: Alan S. Multz, MD. Nassau University Medical Center, 2201 Hempstead Turnpike, East Meadow, NY 11554. (P): 516-572-6501, (F): 516-572-5609, e-mail: amultz@numc.edu, multzman@ optonline.net.

Epidemiology

This is an acquired immune disorder that has its greatest incidence in children. However, in the adult years, this disorder increases in incidence with increasing age. While there is a more female predominance in adults aged < 60, over the age of 60 years the incidence is essentially equal [1]. Although an incidence of 22 million cases per year has been reported, it is likely that this is underestimated since the diagnosis in the prior studies was only made after the patients had symptoms.

Definition

Generally, ITP is defined by one of three groups of patients who have platelet counts less < 100,000/mm^3. Those who are "newly diagnosed", considered to be those diagnosed at time zero to up three months duration. Those who are classified as "persistent", have the diagnosis with them for 3 to 12 months duration. Then there is the group that has "chronic ITP", defined as those who have had the diagnosis for > 12 months duration.

Clincial Presentation

ITP is a disorder that can be characterized by episodes of bleeding that manifests itself with bruising to episodes of bleeding that are more obvious. There can be petechiae or frank purpura in some of the patients. The bleeding episodes are rarely life threatening, so massive GI bleeds or intracranial hemorrhages are uncommon. Bleeding episodes are usually things like gingival bleeding, epistaxis or vaginal bleeding. However, there is considerable variability in how each individual patient can present and some of the rarer bleeding presentations mentioned as noted above can increase in likelihood as age increases [2, 3]. Physical examination findings are common in the oral cavity, the eyes, the skin, GI tract (bleeding detected on examination) or the vagina (for a female patient with vaginal bleeding).

Diagnosis

Primary ITP is a diagnosis that is best made after the many known causes of secondary ITP have been ruled out. It is important to evaluate the patient for some of the secondary causes of ITP. These include testing for both HIV and Hepatitis C, both of which have been associated with secondary ITP.

A more detailed discussion of this will be in the pathophysiology part of this chapter. Systemic lupus erythematosus (SLE) is also a known cause of secondary ITP along with various disturbances in the immune system (lymphoproliferative disorders such as chronic lymphocytic leukemia), the antiphospholipid antibody syndrome and abnormalities in gamma globulin production that manifest with hypogammaglobulinemia. Other infections (beside

HIV and Hepatitis C) have also been known to produce secondary ITP. Other viruses, like varicella (VZV) for example, have also been associated with the development of ITP [4].

There have also been reports of an association between ITP and *Helicobacter pylori* infection, but at best it is fair say to that evidence in support of this is equivocal [5]. There are medications that are that associated with secondary ITP that include quinine, sulfa-containing drugs, Alemtuzumab and purine analogs such as Fludarabine.

Laboratory Testing

The most important laboratory study to make the diagnosis is to do a complete blood count with a platelet count along with examination of the peripheral smear. For example, it is important to note the absence of schistocytes, the presence of which would change the differential diagnosis in patients with thrombocytopenia. Platelet clumping is not an uncommon cause of falsely low platelet counts and may be due to multiple different etiologies such as interaction with the diluent (like EDTA-dependent agglutinins), an inadequate specimen or by the presence of giant platelets.

Interactions with the diluent, as is the case with EDTA may be rectified by using a different anticoagulant as the diluent like heparin or citrate. Cold, either in a patient with a low core body temperature or caused by improper handling of a collected blood specimen may also be a cause of pseudothrombocytopenia. Antibody testing is usually not recommended due to the lack of both specificity and sensitivity in the present assays [6]. Other studies recommended include HIV and Hepatitis C testing, screening serologies for SLE and serum protein electrophoresis with measurement of immunoglobulin levels. Bone marrow aspiration is a controversial issue, but the latest evidence based guidelines regarding the diagnosis of ITP do not recommend that this test be performed [6, 7].

It is more likely to be considered in an elderly patient, > 60 years of age, and is performed to rule out disorders such as a myelodysplastic syndrome or a lymphoproliferative disorder. If the thrombocytopenia is accompanied by anemia, a Coombs test may be helpful in ruling in Evans syndrome, which is a diagnosis of autoimmune hemolytic anemia accompanied by simultaneous ITP.

Differential Diagnosis

The differential diagnosis for ITP is extensive. Pseudothrombocytopenia has been reported with abciximab treatment [8] and the problem of clumping on peripheral smear has already been discussed in the laboratory section of this chapter. Hypersplenism is usually due to the presence of portal hypertension. The most common etiology of this is alcohol related liver disease. The thrombocytopenia is usually mild and due to the pooling of the platelets in the sinusoids of the spleen [9]. It is also important to note that alcohol has a direct toxic effect on the bone marrow that also affects platelet production. There are a series of hereditary thrombocytopenias. They are quite rare but worth including in the discussion. The inheritance patterns for these disorders can be autosomal dominant, autosomal recessive or X-linked. MYH9 gene-related disorders are inherited in an autosomal dominant pattern and include May-Hegglin syndromes as well as other less known syndromes as an example. An example of an autosomal recessive inherited disorder is thrombocytopenia with absent radii syndrome as well as congenital amegakaryocytic thrombocytopenia and Bernard-Soulier syndrome.

Wiskott - Aldrich syndrome represents an example of an X-linked cause of thrombocytopenia with other immune system manifestations which include recurrent infections.

Type 2B von Willebrand disease is transmitted as an autosomal dominant disease. There is increased binding of von Willebrand factor to the circulating platelets and then the platelets are either abnormally cleared or sequestrated [10]. Myelodysplastic syndrome (MDS) may also manifest itself as thrombocytopenia and has been reported to mimic ITP [11].

Many bacteria and viral infections, in addition to the previous mentioned HIV, Hepatitis C and Varicella have also been described to cause ITP. Infections such as Rubella, Cytomegalovirus (CMV), Epstein Barr virus (EBV) and Ehrlichiosis for example have been associated with thrombocytopenia [12]. These infections as well as others can also be associated with disseminated intravascular coagulation (DIC), which not only affects the platelets, but also affects the coagulation system. With DIC, it is not uncommon to have simultaneous disturbances in the coagulation profile along with thrombocytopenia. To rule out this disorder, examination of the peripheral smear is critical along with examining the coagulation profile of the patient. If undiagnosed or misdiagnosed, DIC can lead to death.

Thrombotic thrombocytopenic microangiopathies represent another group of diseases characterized by thrombocytopenia along with microangiopathic hemolytic anemia also associated with microvascular thrombosis. In this disorder, review of the peripheral smear is again essential and generally, these disorders do not involve the coagulation system. DIC can also be included in this group of diseases that includes thrombocytopenic thrombotic purpura (TTP) and hemolytic uremic syndrome (HUS). In TTP, there are five findings that are generally looked for in the patient; these include 1) microangiopathic hemolytic anemia; 2) fever; 3) neurologic findings; 4) renal failure; and 5) thrombocytopenia. We have come to understand that in this disease, all five findings are not required to make a clinical diagnosis nor to initiate empiric treatment if there is significant enough clinical reason. This disease is due to either a lack or the development of antibodies to a specific metalloprotease named ADAMTS13 which is involved in the cleavage of von Willebrand Factor.

HUS is a clinical syndrome that includes microangiopathic hemolytic anemia, renal failure and thrombocytopenia. This disease is more prevalent in children and has been associated with invasive *Escherichia coli* Type 0157:H7 infection.

Heparin-induced thrombocytopenia (HIT) can present clinically in two different ways. The overall incidence of HIT has been reported at about 2.6% with unfractionated heparin (UFH) and 0.2% for low molecular weight heparin (LMWH) [13]. In HIT-1, after exposure to UFH or LMWH, thrombocytopenia will develop characterized by a mild to moderate reduction in the platelet count. This is not felt to be an immunologically mediated process but rather due to direct effect of heparin on platelets. If the platelet count is low enough, the clinical concern is bleeding. HIT-2 (also referred to heparin-induced thrombocytopenia with thrombosis), can be a life threatening problem due to platelet activation and is due to the development of antibodies to platelet factor 4. The frequency of HIT-2 has been noted to be anywhere from 20% to 50% of all HIT cases [14].

Delayed-onset HIT has been described in patients, days after discontinuation of all heparin therapy. The true incidence of this syndrome has not really been well established, but it has been reported that this occurs on the average of nine days after the conclusion of heparin treatment [15]. Calculation of the 4 T's score is recommended as part of the algorithm used in the diagnostic workup fir HIT.

These are 1) thrombocytopenia; 2) timing of the platelet count fall; 3) thrombosis or other sequelae; and 4) other causes for thrombocytopenia [16]. This simple calculation will help determine the likelihood of HIT.

Pathophysiology

The first evidence of the immune mechanism leading to platelet destruction was provided by the Harrington experiments. In 1951 Harrington has infused blood from a patient with ITP into a healthy individual and after two hours he noticed a decrease in platelet count to zero with recovery after few days [17]. Later in 1965 Shulman has demonstrated the immunoglobulin origin of the platelet antibodies [18].

The platelet count is reflecting a balance between platelet production and destruction. The concept that ITP is a disease of increased platelet destruction as well as a disease of decreased platelet production has gained now universal acceptance. Emerging new data are going to change the landscape of first line therapy in patients with ITP in order to change the natural history of the disease with the goal of reducing the number of patients who develop chronic ITP.

The initial sensitizing trigger of the immune process in ITP leading to the production of platelet antibodies is obscure in adult ITP. In childhood ITP infections are thought to be initiating event. The immune process does require an intact reticuloendothelial system. Cells of the reticuloendothelial system will be involved in the phagocytosis of the antibody- platelet complex. These antigen presenting cells (APC) are processing the antigenic proteins into small peptides. APC expressing the platelet specific antigens are implicated in T cell activation leading to antigen specific expansion of B cells. B cells are further involved in the production of glycoprotein specific antibodies. Anti-platelet antibodies are directed against GPIIb/IIIa and GP Ib/IX present on the platelet surface leading to increased platelet destruction, also reflected in a decrease of the normal platelet life span of 7-10 days.

Given the expression of GP IIb/IIIa and GPIb/IX on the developing megakaryocytes the platelet antibodies are also directly involved in impairing megakaryocyte growth maturation and even apoptosis [19]. Other autoantibodies detected in patients with ITP are directed against the thrombopoietin receptor c-Mpl, being directly implicated in suppression of the megakaryopoiesis [20].

Antiplatelet antibodies are nonspecific and present in other autoimmune disorders. They are not present in every patient with ITP suggesting the existence of other mechanisms implicated in the pathogenesis of ITP. Platelets bound by antiplatelet antibodies are further cleared by the macrophages of the reticuloendothelial system via the FCγ receptor.

FCY receptors on the surface of splenic macrophages can be stimulatory and inhibitory. Predisposing polymorphisms in cytokines and FCY receptors has been reported [21, 22]. Other studies describe an imbalance of the activating and inhibitory FCY receptors in ITP patients with a shift to an activating type [23]. T cells play a role in the pathophysiology of ITP. Complex T cell dysregulation includes an increase in the Th1/Th2 ratio consistent with a pro-inflammatory response [24], dysregulation of regulatory T cells [25] and presence of cytotoxic T cells. Th2 cells and regulatory T cells, functioning as suppressors of the immune system are not only reduced in number but also functionally impaired [25].

The increase in cytotoxic T cells is governed by the same stimulatory influence of the Th1 lymphocytes and is directed against platelets and megakaryocytes [26]. After exposure to platelet antibodies, T cells continue to stimulate antibody production.

Although the megakaryocyte number in the bone marrow of patients with ITP seems to be increased and the megakaryocyte appears normal under light microscopy, electronic microscopic studies in fact show significant megakaryocyte damage with vacuolization of the cytoplasm, disruption of borders, increased mitochondrial size and expression of caspase 3 on immunohistochemistry [27]. Platelet production by the bone marrow megakaryocytes is suppressed in ITP.

Thrombopoietin (TPO) is synthesized by the liver at a constant rate, regulated primarily by its clearance and under no translational or post-translational control. TPO is bound to platelets, megakaryocytes and megakaryocyte precursors after release. TPO bound to platelets is being internalized and cleared in conjunction with the platelets. In ITP, there is a rapid clearance and therefore a low circulating TPO. This provides the rationale for the use of TPO agonists in the therapy of ITP. At the same time it does give us the explanation of the failures after splenectomy and other therapies with direct impact on the platelet destruction. TPO agonists bind to the TPO receptor with downstream signaling. The increase in platelet production secondary to TPO agonists makes more platelets available in the peripheral circulation that can be rapidly cleared resulting in an increase in the total platelet count.

Cines et al. [28] describe three mechanisms of immune tolerance defects involved in ITP. Two are defects in peripheral tolerance and then one central defect. The peripheral tolerance defect develops during immune stimulation and differentiation blocks which lead to the development of skewed B cell subtypes. Central tolerance arises during B cell development in the bone marrow or T cell development in the thymus. While the peripheral tolerance problem is considered to be platelet specific and responsive to therapy, the central tolerance problem is less responsive to therapy due to reconstitution of the same autoimmune process after therapy.

Loss of peripheral tolerance is also implicated in ITP secondary to infections Hepatitis C, HIV, *H Pylori*, CMV, VZV and others. Hepatitis C is the most common infection associated with ITP. The pathogenesis of ITP secondary to infections is explained by molecular mimicry and development of cross reactive platelet antibodies. HIV infection is a well described, treatable cause of ITP and additionally infects the megakaryocytes.

Although associated with mild thrombocytopenia, platelet increases in response to bacterial eradication of H Pylori are seen and screening for H Pylori in patients who are candidates for antibacterial therapy are recommended. Failure to correct thrombocytopenia in these patients seems to correlate with the development of antigen independent autoreactive clones [29].

Genetic syndromes provide further insight into the disturbance of central tolerance. Combined variable immunodeficiency (CVID) is associated with a late defect in B cell maturation leading to hypogammaglobulinemia. ITP usually precedes the diagnosis of CVID [30]. The autoimmune lymphoproliferative syndrome, characterized by defective FAS mediated T cell lymphocyte apoptosis due to mutations in genes encoding for FAS or FAS ligand is linked with an accumulation of CD4-/CD8-/CD3+ T cells, lymphadenopathy, splenomegaly and autoimmune cytopenias [30].

Patients with Evans syndrome have involvement of two lineages with thrombocytopenia preceding the development of hemolytic anemia.

There is a clear distinction between antiplatelet antibodies and anti Rh directed red cell antibodies in this entity. Acquired defects in central tolerance include: systemic lupus erythematosus, antiphospholipid antibody syndrome and posttransplant ITP [28].

Who Should Be Treated?

Goal of therapy in ITP is to maintain a hemostatic platelet count with minimal toxicity. While the intent of therapy in ITP is not to normalize the platelet count and just to achieve a hemostatic level, patients with a platelet count less than 30,000/mm^3 require therapy according to all the current guidelines. The only exceptions to this cut off value are patients with active bleeding, patients having an associated platelet dysfunction, patients with coagulation abnormality or on anticoagulation therapy who would benefit from a higher platelet goal of at least 50,000/mm^3. A very important paradigm in ITP is to avoid unnecessary therapy for asymptomatic patients with mild thrombocytopenia.

The International Working Group (IWG) does provide recommendations on target platelet counts before surgical procedures, with close consideration of the emergency of the procedure. The recommendations are: for simple dental extraction a platelet goal of $\geq$ 30,000/ mm^3; for complex dental extraction and minor surgery $\geq$ 50,000/mm^3; for major surgery $\geq$ 80,000/mm^3 and neurosurgery $\geq$ 100,000/mm^3 [31].

In an effort to standardize the reporting of bleeding events in ITP, the IWG is proposing an ITP bleeding assessment tool which grades the severity of bleeding into three main areas: S- skin, M- visible mucosa, O- organs. The severity of bleeding can be graded from 1-4, 5 being reported as fatal, and the worst bleeding manifestations to be reported at each site. The SMOG system facilitates a uniform reporting of bleeding manifestations in ITP [32].

An compensatory increase in young, large, functionally very active platelets in patients with ITP is an explanation of the lower bleeding manifestations in patients with ITP compared to secondary thrombocytopenias [33]. Greene et al. [34] provides evidence of a better correlation of bleeding manifestations with thromboelastometry and measurements of immature platelet fraction when compared to platelet count or mean platelet volume (MPV).

Initial Therapy in ITP

While therapy in ITP continues to evolve, the production of high affinity platelet specific antibodies over time is providing the rationale for early intervention with immunosuppression with the goal of reducing the number of patients who go on to develop chronic ITP.

By all guidelines, steroids remain the first line therapy in ITP [7, 31]. Steroids diminish platelet destruction and at the same time increase platelet production. They should be administered with caution in patients with relative a contraindication to steroids like those with diabetes, psychiatric disorders, and uncontrolled hypertension.

Intravenous immunoglobulin (IVIG) and anti-D should be used as first line therapy in patients with a contraindication to steroids. Steroid therapy does not change the natural history of the disease associated with initial high response rates, since these responses are not sustained after tapering.

Non-responders to initial therapy should prompt further workup to rule out other causes of thrombocytopenia, like infectious, autoimmune conditions or occult malignancies. The American Society of Hematology (ASH) 2011 ITP guidelines recommend a longer initial course of steroids, prednisone at a dose of 1 mg/kg orally for 3 weeks with a slow taper [7].

Responses to steroids start within a few days with maximal responses in up to 2 weeks of therapy. Steroid dependence is defined by the IWG as an ongoing requirement for corticosteroids for more then 2 months in order to maintain a platelet count above 30,000/ mm^3 and/or to avoid bleeding [35].

The first data on high dose Decadron as initial therapy in ITP were provided by the work of Cheng in 2003 [36]. The 85% response rates noted initially were associated with only 50% sustained responses at 6 month. Italian investigators in GIMEMA [37] did report on two different schedules of high dose Decadron: the first consisted of Decadron 40 mg pulses for 4 days every 28 days for 6 cycles and the second consisted of Decadron 40 mg for 4 days every 14 days for 4 cycles. A 74% response rate at 8 months with these high dose Decadron schedules were published in this trial.

A multicenter phase III trial comparing high dose Decadron to conventional prednisone in patients with ITP based on a 1:1 design did show similar initial response rates with the two regimens, with 19.7% of patients experiencing a sustained response after a single course of Decadron [38]. This trial did not establish the superiority of high dose Decadron.

Inbach was the first to use and observe the efficacy of IVIG in the therapy of two children with immunodeficiency and observed an increase in platelet count [39]. IVIG can be administered in order to augment the response to steroids or in cases of contraindication to steroid use. The recommended dose of IVIG is 1 g/kg as a onetime dose or 0.4 g/kg/day for 5 days. IVIG can be repeated every 10-21 days as necessary. Responses to IVIG are very fast, usually within the first 24 hours. IVIG up regulates the inhibitory FCYIIB receptor on the surface of the splenic phagocytic cells [40].

Side effects to IVIG include acute renal failure, hemolysis and thrombosis. Concomitant use of steroids can decrease the infusion related reactions and aseptic meningitis of IVIG. After an outbreak of Hepatitis C reported in 1993-1995 attributed to a single preparation of IVIG, no further cases of HIV, Hepatitis C or HTLV-1 have been reported [41].

Long term immunomodulatory effects of IVIG are supported by the observation that children treated with IVIG at diagnosis were less likely to develop chronic ITP [42].

Intravenous anti-D interacts with the activating FCYRIIA and FCYRIIIA receptors on the surface of the splenic macrophages [40]. Immune clearance of RBC's coated with anti-D compete for the Fc receptor on the splenic macrophages, minimizing the removal of antibody coated platelets. An intravenous dose of 50-75 micrograms/kg over 3-5 minutes can be used in Rh positive, non-splenectomized patients. A Coombs test should be performed prior to initiation of therapy. Anti-D treatment is contraindicated in patients who are Coombs positive or have hemoglobin levels < 10 g/dl.

Responses to therapy are expected within one week. Duration of platelet response to anti-D is comparable to the response to IVIG. In 2010 the FDA issued a black box warning concerning severe hemolytic reactions. Serious hemolysis may be anticipated in 1 out of 1115 patients [43]. The incidence of hemolysis is higher in patients with renal dysfunction, recent infections like EBV, age more than 65 or a prior history of hemolysis.

The ASH 2011 ITP guidelines recommend the use of anti-D in non-splenectomized patients with close monitoring for hemolysis.

Given the fact that long term responses to first line therapy are modest, investigators are moving the immunomodulatory agents upfront in the therapy of ITP. The first prospective trial to report on the efficacy of upfront Rituximab therapy in patients with ITP was reported by Zaya et al. [44]. 103 patients were randomized to Decadron 40 mg orally for four days versus the same dose of Decadron in combination with Rituximab 375 mg/m^2 weekly for 4 weeks. Patients not responding to Decadron could be salvaged with the Decadron and Rituximab combination. The trial reported 6 month sustained responses in 63% of the Decadron and Rituximab combination treatment group vs. 36% of he Decadron only treatment group (p=0.004, {95%CI} 0.079-0.455). The Decadron and Rituximab combination was able to salvage 56% of patients in the Decadron only arm.

In 2013, Danish investigators reported on an open label phase 3 trial of upfront Rituximab with Decadron vs. Decadron in newly diagnosed patients with ITP with up to 4 years of follow up [45]. This study did confirm the 6 month data from the previous mentioned trial of Zaya's with 58% response rates in the Rituximab with Decadron arm vs. 37% response rates in the Decadron only arm and did demonstrate a longer time to relapse in the combination arm at 4 years. Increased response rates were seen at the expense of increased toxicity. Persistently low IgM levels after 2 years were seen in the Rituximab arm. Although there was no increased rate of infection, long term safety data are currently unknown.

Second Line Therapy in ITP

Rituximab

The sequence of treatments in the second line setting is not well established. The field continues to evolve. ASH 2011 ITP guidelines place Rituximab after splenectomy in patients with an unfavorable response to splenectomy. At the same time the IWG is recommending both Rituximab and splenectomy as treatment options without expressing a stronger recommendation for one versus the other. Rituximab is still not FDA approved for the therapy of ITP, but is widely used by hematologists for this indication.

Rituximab targets CD-20 on the B cell, and impairs autoantibody production. These autoantibodies are platelet specific and directed against GPIIb/IIIa on the platelet surface and on megakaryocytes. The immediate effect of Rituximab on the B cell is an explanation of the rapid platelet recovery seen in patients who have a response. Rituximab also seems to have effects on the T cell component. Its effect contributes to the restoration of the Th1/Th2 ratio [46] and increases the function and number of regulatory T cells [47]. While analyzing the splenectomy specimen in non-responders, Audia et al. [48] found an increase in splenic effector memory CD8+ T cells, leading to an enhanced cytotoxic T cell mediated cell destruction. These CD8+ T cells were not found in the peripheral blood of non-responders, further underlining the importance of the spleen in the process of platelet destruction. Mehevas does explain the lack of response to Rituximab as being due to the persistence of splenic plasma cells and memory B cells [49]. The inclusion of splenectomized and non-splenectomized patients in clinical trials makes it difficult to draw a definite conclusion regarding the best indication for its use. The last meta-analysis of Rituximab before splenectomy was published in 2012 by the French investigators [50].

In order to find an answer as to the place of Rituximab therapy in patients with ITP, while not comparing splenectomy to Rituximab, the meta-analysis reports overall response rates of 57%(95%CI: 48-65) for non-splenectomized patients after Rituximab, complete responses of 41%(95% CI:0.33-0.55). In contradistinction to other studies, the duration of ITP did not have an effect on response rates and on complete responses.

However outcomes with Rituximab therapy at 5 years drop to 20-26% long term responses [49]. Long term responses correlate with a complete response to therapy compared to patients achieving only partial responses. Patients undergoing splenectomy relapse quicker than those who are non-splenectomized. Patients, who respond initially to Rituximab for one year and relapse, will respond to retreatment, while patients achieving a partial response to Rituximab are less likely to respond to retreatment [51].

At ASH 2013 Bussell et al. did report on the combination of Rituximab with three cycles of high dose Decadron [52]. Long term responses similar to splenectomy were seen in patients with ITP of less than 2 years duration. 59% of the responding patients did maintain the response without relapse at 67 months, suggesting that with the addition of high dose Decadron to Rituximab more sustained remissions can be obtained. The rational of this good response is provided by the dual blockade of the B cells and the plasma cells with the combination of Rituximab and Decadron. Rituximab maintenance in a small case series by Mahler et al. in patients with ITP and Evans syndrome seems to be safe in patients relapsing after an initial response to Rituximab therapy [53].

Starting with the working hypothesis that the B cell number is much lower in ITP than in lymphoma, Zaja [54] tested the efficacy of low dose Rituximab at a dose of 100 mg weekly for 4 weeks in patients with ITP. There were significant differences noted between the two dose schedules with a longer median time to response of 35 days in the low dose arm and a shorter duration of response, suggesting that low dose Rituximab activity is moderate during long term follow up.

Hepatitis B (HB) reactivation and the occurrence of progressive multi-focal leukoencephalopathy (PML) are included in the Rituximab black box warning. A HB panel should be ordered on every patient considered a candidate for this treatment. The first prospective study of HB reactivation in patients with diffuse large B cell lymphomas treated with RCHOP by Niitsu et al. [55] brought to our attention HB reactivation in HBsAg negative patients which are also anti-HBc positive. While the reactivation rate in HBsAg positive patients in the pre-Rituxan era was 48%, in HBsAg negative patients the reactivation is 12%. Currently close serial monitoring of HBV DNA levels during therapy, at the end of therapy and 12 months after completion of therapy as well as prophylactic antiviral therapy is part of the standard of care for these patients.

Several cases of PML have been reported at a median time of 5.5 months from the last dose of Rituximab, with 90% mortality and a median time to death of 2 months [56]. PML seem to be more common in certain pathologies with a predisposition to PML, like rheumatoid arthritis and SLE but is less common in ITP. Early diagnosis and attempts to augment immune reconstitution are potential therapies for this severe illness.

Immunizations should be administered before Rituximab therapy, as responses to vaccines are reduced for 4-6 months until the B cells return to their baseline level.

Since the advent of the addition of thrombopoietin receptor antagonists (TPO-RA) and Rituximab to the treatment in ITP patients, the use of other second line immunosuppressive agents has decreased.

The ASH 2011 guidelines due not provide any recommendations on other second line therapies given lack of sufficient evidence based recommendations. IWG lists these medications in alphabetical order, with the intent not to show any preference for one drug over another drug: azathioprine, (a purine inhibitor); cyclosporine, cyclophosphamide (a calcineurin inhibitor and an alkylating agent); danazol (a weak androgen); dapsone; and mycophenolate mofetil (an anti proliferative immunosuppressant). Rituximab and TPO-RA follow at the end of this alphabetical list.

Splenectomy

Splenectomy removes a major site of platelet destruction as well as a major site of antibody production. There is no consensus regarding the indication for splenectomy. Evidence supporting the delay of splenectomy for 6-12 months after diagnosis is based on the potential spontaneous remissions of the disease and responses to first line or second line therapy like Rituximab or TPO-RA, which are used to spare one from splenectomy. IVIG and steroids are used in patients prior to splenectomy to increase platelet counts up to 50,000/mm^3. IVIG has the advantage of not exposing patients in the perioperative period to wound healing problems. Responses to splenectomy are reported in 85% of patients, with 60-65% having long term remissions, thus providing evidence for the best long term results in patients with ITP [57]. 10-20% of patients might achieve partial responses that permit a decrease in use of adjunctive medications and allow maintenance of a hemostatic platelet count.

Patients relapsing after splenectomy are considered to have refractory ITP. Most of the relapses are seen within the first 2 years after splenectomy. A relapse after splenectomy should take into account the possibility of an accessory spleen. Absence of Howell- Jolly bodies on the peripheral smear should alert us to take an accessory spleen into consideration. The possibility of an accessory spleen as a reason for relapse is very low in patients who did not have a response to the initial splenectomy [58].

The international consensus report on investigation and management of ITP considers indium labeled autologous platelet scanning as the most sensitive predictor of responses to splenectomy [59], with previous platelet increase to steroids or IVIG having a very low predictive value.

While ASH is recommending splenectomy over other second line therapies (grade 1B evidence), The IWG equally endorses splenectomy and other therapies, like Rituximab and TPO-RA. Splenectomy does not impair the response to other second line therapies like Rituximab or TPO-RA, the only exception being anti-D therapy.

The mechanism of action of anti-D is based on the competition of anti-D with the FCY receptor on the splenic macrophages.

Boyle et al. [60] reported on splenectomy complications in 1762 patients undergoing splenectomy, out of 9976 patients with the diagnosis of ITP. Both early and late venous thromboembolic events (VTE) were seen in patients after splenectomy, 4.3% vs. 1.7% in patients who did not undergo the procedure, with HR 5.2[CI 3.2-8.5] for early and HR 2.7 [CI

1.9-3.8] for late VTE. The incidence of thromboembolic complications in patients with splenectomy and thalassemia is much higher up to 8.3%, given the increased hypercoagulable state seen in patients with thalassemia [61].

Acute abdominal arterial thrombosis is considered a known surgical complication after abdominal surgery and did occur with a HR 5.4 [CI 2.3-12.5] in the early postoperative period, explaining its lack of occurrence in the late postoperative period. Vascular complications after splenectomy are very complex and can be explained by alterations of the vascular endothelium secondary to accumulation of damaged cells which have been released into the circulation, while the splenic filter is lost, leading to hypercoagulability [62]. The incidence of sepsis reported by Boyle et al. [60] was 11%, compared to 10% of patients who did not undergo this surgical procedure. In 2010, the CDC recommends pneumococcal and meningococcal vaccination and for those with no contraindication, one dose of Haemophilus b vaccination 14 days prior to the procedure. Patients undergoing Rituximab therapy prior to splenectomy might have an impaired antibody response to vaccination, for at least 6 months after Rituximab therapy [63]. These patients should be vaccinated before Rituximab therapy as a lack of response to the standard vaccination 14 days prior to splenectomy can be anticipated. Enteric pathogens are mainly involved in early infections after splenectomy [64]. Patients should be counseled on the use of a medical alert bracelet.

A preoperative platelet count of at least 20,000/mm^3 would be optimal before splenectomy [65], in order to prevent postoperative complications. ASH is recommending either open splenectomy or a laparoscopic approach. Laparoscopic splenectomy does have the same results in cases of accessory spleens [66].

In the postoperative state close follow up is indicated with antibiotic prophylaxis until the critical postoperative period is completed along with thromboprophylaxis, early mobilization, gradual tapering of steroids or TPO-RA in case they have been used as a bridge to splenectomy. Pneumococcal vaccination is to be administered every 5 years in conjunction with annual flu vaccines.

Splenic artery embolization is a modern approach to patients at high risk from or with contraindications to surgical splenectomy [67].

Thrombopoietin Receptor Agonists (TPO-RA)

In the last decades, the introduction of TPO-RA has changed the landscape of ITP. Two TPO-RA agents are currently available for the treatment of patients with an insufficient response to corticosteroids, IVIG or splenectomy.

Eltrombopag is the first oral non-peptide TPO-RA, a small molecule, increasing platelet production by binding to the transmembrane domain of the TPO receptor and not competing with TPO [68]. Eltrombopag dosing starts at 50 mg once daily, with the dose to be titrated based on the platelet response with the goal to achieve and maintain a platelet count $\geq$ 50,000/mm^3 as needed to reduce the risk of bleeding.

Eltrombopag should be administered on an empty stomach and at least 4 hours apart from food, medications or other supplements. Romiplostim is a fusion protein combining an Fc fragment to four identical peptides and binds to the TPO receptor [69].

In contradistinction to Romiplostim, Eltrombopag does not compete with the circulating TPO for receptor binding. Romiplostim is dosed subcutaneous initially at 1 microgram/kg once weekly with adjustments of the dose by 1 microgram/kg increments to achieve a platelet count≥ 50,000/mm^3 and to reduce the risk of bleeding. Lack of response to one TPO-RA does not imply a lack of efficacy to the other TPO-RA.

The RAISE study, a phase III, double blind, placebo-controlled randomized trial, allocated patients with ITP of 6 months duration to Eltrombopag therapy for 6 months versus standard of care. A platelet increase was noticed in 79% of the patients in the Eltrombopag arm, compared to 28% in the standard of care arm [70]. Patients responded to Eltrombopag irrespective of splenectomy status. Serious bleeding was observed in 7% of patients in the placebo arm and <1% in the Eltrombopag arm. 7% of patients in the Eltrombopag arm did experience mild increase in liver enzymes, compared to 2% in the placebo arm. The incidence of thromboembolic events was 2% in the Eltrombopag arm. Long term safety and efficacy of Eltrombopag for treatment of chronic ITP is reflected in the ongoing EXTEND study [71]. An interim analysis after 3 years of this study enrolled 299 patients splenectomized and non-splenectomized, with ITP of more than 6 months duration. 85% of the patients achieved a platelets≥ 50,000 mm^3 at least once on therapy regardless of their splenectomy status. An associated 50% decrease in bleeding symptoms including clinically significant bleeding (WHO grade 2-4) was noted, with a constant response over time illustrated by the stable dose of medication throughout the treatment.

Safety parameters did reveal rare, mild and reversible hepatic dysfunction, a low incidence of bone marrow fibrosis, no increase in cataracts or hematologic malignancies.5% of the patients did experience arterial and venous thromboembolic events, half of them at a platelet count below normal range.

An update on the EXTEND study with 6 year data was presented at the ASH meeting in 2013. Longer follow up did not reveal an increase in side effects, but continued to demonstrate a sustained increase in platelets and reduced bleeding [72].

An open label trial did randomize patients before splenectomy (n=234) with the intent of delaying or sparing splenectomy to Romiplostim for 52 weeks or standard of care therapy, based on the investigators institutional guidelines. The platelet response in the Romiplostim arm was higher compared to the standard of care arm. Patients in the Romiplostim arm had fewer splenectomies, lower transfusion requirements and fewer bleeding episodes [73]. The concluding results from an international, multi-center single arm study evaluating efficacy and safety of Romiplostim, the largest prospective study in adult ITP, reported 90% response rates to Romiplostim, independent of splenectomy status. No neutralizing antibodies were found and side effects like bone marrow fibrosis, hemorrhage and thromboembolic events were each observed in 0.5% of patients [74].

While TPO-RA are being perceived as long term treatments, case studies of remissions after cessation of Romiplostim have been reported [75]. Further studies are underway to validate this very important finding. A possible explanation of this response relies on the immune process, involving an increase in the number and activity of regulatory T cells, regulatory B cells as well as NK cells.

Ghadaki et al. [76] documented a decline of anti-GP IIb/IIIa antibodies in one patient while on TPO-RA therapy. Results of a French observational study by Mehevas et al. did report that, 15% of 54 patients were in remission with stable platelet counts while off the TPO-RA. Patients on Romiplostim and Eltrombopag were included in this study [77].

Data on the use of TPO-RA in ITP of less than six months duration is starting to emerge. Almaguer et al. [78] reported on results in patients with newly diagnosed ITP treated with

Decadron 40 mg orally for 4 days and Eltrombopag 50 mg orally days 5-32. At 6 months, 50% of patients had platelet counts above 100,000/mm^3 and 25% between 30,000/mm^3 and 100,000/mm^3 with a relapse free survival at one year being 66.7%.

TPO-RA agents used upfront in steroid refractory bleeding patients, work faster then other second line immunosuppressive agents, at the same time sparing the patient the immunosuppressive toxicity of these medications [79].

Refractory ITP

Refractory ITP is defined by IWG as ITP relapsing after splenectomy or failing splenectomy, which might also have a continuous need to use adjunctive measures to achieve a hemostatic platelet count. Refractory ITP also requires the exclusion of any causes of secondary ITP, like drug induced ITP, hereditary thrombocytopenia or a myelodysplastic syndrome as examples. Given the decline in patients undergoing splenectomies, the number of patients in this category is falling. ASH 2011 ITP guidelines endorse a platelet goal of 30,000/mm^3 in nonbleeding patients with refractory ITP and is recommending against any effort to increase the platelets above this platelet number. Patients with platelet countless then 30,000/mm^3 have an increased risk of bleeding related mortality, 36.7% and 6.7% died with treatment related complications [80].

Patients with refractory ITP maintain some response to on demand doses of steroids and IVIG. The intention is to obtain hemostatic platelet counts in these patients during preoperative situations and bleeding. Different multi-agent combinations have been studied. The rational behind multi-agent combinations is the use of different therapies with different mechanisms of action with non overlapping toxicity profiles. A case series reported by Burchov et al. [81] used a four drug combination of IVIG, methylprednisolone, vinca alkaloids and anti-D with subsequent maintenance with azathioprine and danazol, with two thirds of patients on maintenance accomplishing a platelet count of 50,000/mm^3 without other treatments. Arnold et al. [82] reported on the combination of azathioprine, cyclosporine and mycophenolate mofetil with good results. The Cyclosporine- Romiplostim-IVIG combination [83] is based on the combination of T cell inhibition by cyclosporine, increased platelet production by TPO-RA and decreased platelet destruction by IVIG. In practice, with the availability of TPO-RA with high response rates, independent of the presence or absence of the spleen, fewer patients are being treated with these combination regimens.

What Second Line Therapy Should I Choose?

The treating physician is challenged by the question of which therapy to use in the second line setting. Is there a preferred or optimal second line therapy in patients with ITP? There is no consensus between available guidelines about the best second line therapy. Splenectomy was once the gold standard and preferred in 50-60% of patients.

The incidence has decreased to 20-25% [4]. Due to the lack of randomized studies comparing medical second line treatment options to splenectomy, as well as to each other, the recommendations for the second line setting need to be individualized. These decisions must take into account the risks and benefits of every therapeutic option.

The goal of patient counseling is to empower the patient to play an active role in the treatment decision and to provide adequate medical information to support the decision.

Rituximab has response rates of 40-60%, complete responses at 3-5 years being much lower at 20%. The recent trials combining high dose Decadron with Rituximab are challenging these results, claiming response rates similar to splenectomy. Side effects to Rituximab are infusion related reactions, hypogammaglobulinemia and the risk of viral reactivation, like reactivation of HB and rarely of Jacob Creutzfeldt (JC). TPO-RA agonists have 60-90% response rates. They cannot be used as a sole therapy in emergency situations, since responses are expected after 1-2 weeks of therapy, but they could have a supplementary role in management of ITP emergencies. A small number of patients fail to maintain a response once a stable platelet count has been obtained [85].

Rebound thrombocytopenia upon interruption of these medications has been very well described. The indefinite duration of therapy with TPO-RA makes compliance a very important problem to be taken into consideration when making a therapy decision. While being approved in Europe only for patients after splenectomy failures, in the US, the recommendations are independent of the presence or absence of the spleen.

However, at present, long term safety data beyond five years are not available on this treatment. Eltrombopag has a black box warning regarding hepatic toxicity and liver function tests should be monitored every 1-2 months during therapy. The risk of bone marrow fibrosis is low. A bone marrow biopsy at the beginning of therapy as an assessment of the baseline marrow is not needed prior to starting TPO-RA. Bone marrow biopsies can be considered in patients when there is a loss of response to TPO-RA, or in any case of a change in the peripheral smear.

The risk to induce malignancies and MDS during therapy is also low, but the concern of progression to AML during therapy for thrombocytopenia in MDS patients does exist, making the TPO-RA not to be used in these patients. The risk of arterial and venous thrombosis is not trivial. Almost all patients who developed VTE in clinical trials had pre-existing thrombotic risk factors, although patients with a history of deep venous thrombosis and severe vascular disease were not included in these studies. The recommendations are to use the lowest possible dose to maintain a platelet count of 50,000/mm^3. Administration of aspirin is recommended for platelet counts above 50,000/mm^3.

Given the rate of spontaneous remissions in patients with ITP after 1-2 years after initial diagnosis, all the mentioned treatments can be used as a bridge to splenectomy if necessary. It is still not clear when splenectomy is advisable as a next step. While still associated with the most durable remissions, responses to splenectomy are not easily predictable. Splenectomy involves surgical related mortality and morbidity as well as infectious and thromboembolic complications.

ITP in Pregnancy

When compared to women with a previous diagnosis of ITP, women with a new diagnosis of ITP during pregnancy are more likely to require therapy during pregnancy [86].

The outcome of newborns of mothers with ITP is good, with a mortality of less than 1% [87]. A platelet goal of 20,000-30,000/mm^3 has been established to be safe during pregnancy [88]. While remaining stable throughout the pregnancy, platelets are more likely to drop during the third trimester, requiring frequent monitoring as delivery is approaching.

Steroids are the first line therapy in patients with ITP during pregnancy. The recommendations are to start at a low dose of prednisone 10 mg orally. Considered safe in pregnancy, steroids are also associated with side effects. In pregnant women, these can be an increase in weight, high glucose levels, and hypertension as well as in the newborn, with an increased incidence in oral cleft palate [89]. IVIG can be used in order to augment the platelet count if needed and is considered safe in pregnancy. The ASH 2011 guidelines do not comment on the use of anti-D therapy. IWG recommends anti-D at 50-75 micrograms/kg during the second and third trimester. Anti-D does cross the placenta and the newborns need to be monitored for hemolysis. The beneficial effect of steroids given before 34 weeks of gestation to improve lung maturation prior to a premature delivery is confirmed by a meta-analysis by Roberts D et al. [90].

Patients with a suboptimal result to first line therapy can be considered for combination therapy of high dose steroids of 1000 mg methyl-prednisolone and IVIG. Second line therapies used in nonpregnant women are rarely considered for pregnant women due to safety concerns. Azathioprine and cyclosporine A seem to be safe in pregnancy but are rarely used. The use of Rituximab is also limited given the same concerns.

During delivery, the ASH guidelines state that bleeding complications are not related to the degree of thrombocytopenia, with no differences in bleeding between caesarian sections (C-section) and vaginal delivery thus concluding that the delivery of patients with ITP should be based on obstetric recommendations only [7]. ITP in pregnancy is not an indication for C-section. This recommendation is based on the lack of evidence defining a safe platelet count in the antepartum and postpartum period. Vaginal deliveries in patients with a platelet count as low as 19,000/mm^3 have been reported [84]. Given the potential need of conversion of a vaginal delivery to a C-section, the IWG recommends a platelet goal of 50,000/mm^3 [31]. The high risk of bleeding and the severe implications of a spinal hematoma during epidural anesthesia indicate the need for higher platelet counts of 75,000-100,000/mm^3 prior to this procedure by obstetric anesthetists. A short term course of one to two weeks of steroids and doses of IVIG can be used in preparation for epidural anesthesia.

25% of the newborns of mothers with ITP are thrombocytopenic. The rate of associated bleeding complications for newborns is low [91]. Measurement of fetal platelet count by periumbilical or fetal scalp vein sampling carries a bleeding risk and is not recommended on routine basis. The highest risk of newborn bleeding can be predicted by a history of a previous delivery with this complication [92].

In this situation a C-section could be recommended [93].

Given the lack of safety data for Rituximab, TPO-RA and other second line immunosuppressant agents, splenectomy is an option for refractory cases. In practice splenectomy is rarely performed. The timing of splenectomy should also take into consideration the risks involved dependent on the age of gestation. While splenectomy poses a risk of accelerated premature labor during the first trimester, after 20 weeks of gestation the risks are related to the size of the pregnant uterus [94]. Currently there is evidence available that women with ITP in remission after splenectomy are at risk of relapse during pregnancy.

Mothers after splenectomy might be able to maintain a stable platelet count while the newborn could experience thrombocytopenia [95].

Secondary ITP in the context of antiphospholipid syndrome is treated in similar fashion as in nonpregnant women, and there is an increased risk of thrombosis in these patients [96]. Low dose aspirin is being used in patients with a positive lupus anticoagulant or positive anticardiolipin antibodies in the absence of a history of thromboembolism when platelet count is above 50,000/mm^3. Patients with history of spontaneous miscarriages or previous thrombosis are candidates for low molecular weight heparin, considered to be safe if platelets are above 50,000/mm^3. Pregnancy is a hypercoagulable state and despite thrombocytopenia patients should be considered for DVT prophylaxis.

Emergency Bleeding in ITP

Bleeding patients with ITP continue to remain a challenge for physicians. IVIG has the fastest response with an expected increase in platelet count within 24 hours. Combination regimens of high dose steroids and IVIG are used in conjunction with platelet transfusion every 8 hours [97]. Although the transfused platelets are destroyed, they still have a beneficial hemostatic effect in the bleeding patients. Platelet survival can be increased if platelets are transfused after the infusion of IVIG. From the second line options the IWG is reporting on rapid responses of combinations containing steroids, IVIG, anti-D and Vincristine [98]. Limited data are available in the literature regarding recombinant factor VII. A proposed mechanism of action of recombinant factor VII is the direct activation of platelets as well as the activation of factor X, with thrombin formation on the activated platelet surface, leading to further enhancement of platelet function [99]. Studies using recombinant factor VII in children report a 4.3% incidence of thrombotic events [100]. Adjunctive measures to control mucosal bleeding like ε-aminocaproic acid and tranexamic acid, inhibitors of fibrinolysis can be used. The only exception is patients with hematuria, who could develop thrombi in the renal pelvis and ureters while on antifibrinolytic therapy.

Conclusion

Steroids, IVIG and anti-D remain first line therapy in ITP. New data on the use of Rituximab and TPO-RA are emerging. The decision of therapy in second line setting needs to be individualized, while balancing pros and cons of splenectomy, Rituximab and TPO-RA. Splenectomy has the highest cure rate and because of spontaneous remissions and improvement up to one year in ITP, should be considered in ITP nonresponsive after one year of medical therapy, in the chronic phase of the disease. The long term responses with Rituximab are low, 20% at 5 years. TPO-RA have good response rates in 80-90% of patients, with unknown long term side effects beyond 5 years, requiring compliance and few patients might maintain responses after their discontinuation.

References

[1] Frederiksen, H., Schmidt, K. The incidence of idiopathic thrombocytopenic purpura in adults increases with age. *Blood* 1999; 94: 909.

[2] Cortelazzo, S., Finazzi, G., Buelli, M., Molteni, A., Viero, P., Barbui, T. High risk of severe bleeding in aged patients with chronic idiopathic thrombocytopenic purpura. *Blood*. 1991;77(1):31.

[3] Guthrie, T. H. Jr, Brannan, D. P., Prisant, L. M. Idiopathic thrombocytopenic purpura in the older adult patient. *Am. J. Med. Sci.* 1988;296(1):17.

[4] Wright, J. F., Blanchette, V. S., Wang, H., Arya, N., Petric, M., Semple, J. W., Chia, W. K., Freedman, J. Characterization of platelet-reactive antibodies in children with varicella-associated acute immune thrombocytopenic purpura (ITP). *Br. J. Haematol.* 1996; 95(1):145.

[5] Arnold, D. M., Bernotas, A., Nazi, I., Stasi, R., Kuwana, M., Liu, Y., Kelton, J. G., Crowther, M. A. Platelet count response to H. pylori treatment in patients with immune thrombocytopenic purpura with and without H. pylori infection: a systematic review. *Haematologica*. 2009; 94(6):850.

[6] George, J. N., Woolf, S. H., Raskob, G. E., Wasser, J. S., Aledort, L. M., Ballem, P. J., Blanchette, V. S., Bussel, J. B., Cines, D. B., Kelton, J. G., Lichtin, A. E., McMillan, R., Okerbloom, J. A., Regan, D. H., Warrier, I. Idiopathic thrombocytopenic purpura: a practice guideline developed by explicit methods for the American Society of Hematology. *Blood*. 1996; 88(1):3.

[7] Neunert, C., Lim, W., Crowther, M., Cohen, A., Solberg, L. Jr, Crowther, M. A., American Society of Hematology. The American Society of Hematology 2011 evidence-based practice guideline for immune thrombocytopenia. *Blood*. 2011; 117 (16):4190.

[8] Sane, D. C., Damaraju, L. V., Topol, E. J., Cabot, C. F., Mascelli, M. A., Harrington, R. A., Simoons, M. L., Califf, R. M. Occurrence and clinical significance of pseudothrombocytopenia during abciximab therapy. *J. Am. Coll. Cardiol.* 2000; 36(1): 75.

[9] Aster, R. H. Pooling of platelets in the spleen: role in the pathogenesis of "hypersplenic" thrombocytopenia. *J. Clin. Invest.* 1966; 45(5):645.

[10] Ruggeri, Z. M., Pareti, F. I., Mannucci, P. M., Ciavarella, N., Zimmerman, T. S. Heightened interaction between platelets and factor VIII/von Willebrand factor in a new subtype of von Willebrand's disease. *N. Engl. J. Med.* 1980; 302(19):1047.

[11] Menke, D. M., Colon-Otero, G., Cockerill, K. J., Jenkins, R. B., Noel, P., Pierre, R. V. Refractory thrombocytopenia. A myelodysplastic syndrome that may mimic immune thrombocytopenic purpura. *Am. J. Clin. Pathol.* 1992; 98(5):502.

[12] Stasi, R., Willis, F., Shannon, M. S., Gordon-Smith, E. C. Infectious causes of chronic immune thrombocytopenia. *Hematol. Oncol. Clin. North Am.* 2009; 23(6):1275.

[13] Martel, N., Lee, J., Wells, P. S. Risk for heparin-induced thrombocytopenia with unfractionated and low-molecular-weight heparin thromboprophylaxis: a meta-analysis. *Blood*. 2005; 106(8):2710.

[14] Linkins, L. A., Dans, A. L., Moores, L. K., Bona, R., Davidson, B. L., Schulman, S., Crowther, M., American College of Chest Physicians. *Treatment and prevention of*

heparin-induced thrombocytopenia: Antithrombotic Therapy and Prevention of Thrombosis, 9th ed: American College of Chest Physicians Evidence-Based Clinical Practice Guidelines. *Chest.* 2012; 141(2 Suppl.):e495S.

[15] Warkentin, T. E., Kelton, J. G. Delayed-onset heparin-induced thrombocytopenia and thrombosis. *Ann. Intern. Med.* 2001; 135(7):502.

[16] Lo, G. K., Juhl, D., Warkentin, T. E., Sigouin, C. S., Eichler, P., Greinacher, A. Evaluation of pretest clinical score (4 T's) for the diagnosis of heparin-induced thrombocytopenia in two clinical settings. *J. Thromb. Haemost.* 2006; 4(4):759.

[17] Harrington, W. J., Sprague, C. C., Minnich, V., Moonre, C. V., Aulvin, R. C., Dubach, R. Immunologic mechanism in idiopathic and neonatal thrombocytopenic purpura. *Ann. Intern. Med.* 1953; 38(3):433-462.

[18] Shulman, N. R., Marder, V. J., Weinrach, R. S. Similarities between known antiplatelet antibodies and the factor responsible for thrombocytopenia in idiopathic purpura. Physiologic, serologic and isotopic studies. *Ann. N Y Acad. Sci.* 1965; 124(2):499-542.

[19] Toltl, L. J., Nazi, I., Jafari, R., Arnold, D. M. Piecing together the humoral and cellular mechanism of immune thrombocytopenia. *Semin. Thromb. Hemost.* 2011; 37(6):631-639.

[20] Kuwana, M., Okazaki, Y., Kajihara, M., et al. Antibody to c-Mpl (thrombopoietin receptor) in systemic lupus erythematosus: relationship to thrombocytopenia with megakaryocytic hypoplasia. *Arthritis Rheum.* 2002; 46(8):2148-2159.

[21] Foster, C. B., Zhu, S., Erichsen, H. C., et al. Polymorphisms in inflammatory cytokines and Fcgamma receptors in childhood chronic immune thrombocytopenic purpura: a pilot study. *Br. J. Haematol.* 2001; 113:596-599.

[22] Breunis, W. B., van Mirre, E., Bruin, M., Geissler, J., de Boer, M., Peters, M., Roos, D., de Haas, M., Koene, H. R., Kuijpers, T. W. Copy number variation of the activating FCGR2C gene predisposes to idiopathic thrombocytopenic purpura. *Blood* 2008; 111: 1029-1038.

[23] Liu, X., Ma, S., Sun, J., Ren, J., Shi, Y., Sun, L., Dong, X., Qin, P., Guo, S., Hou, M., Peng, J. High-dose dexamethasone shifts the balance of stimulatory and inhibitory Fcγ receptors on monocytes in patients with primary immune thrombocytopenia. *Blood* 2011; 117:2061-2069.

[24] Semple, J. W., Milev, Y., Cosgrave, D., Mody, M., Hornstein, A., Blanchette, V., Freedman, J. Differences in serum cytokine levels in acute and chronic autoimmune thrombocytopenic purpura: relationship to platelet phenotype and antiplatelet T-cell reactivity. *Blood* 1996; 87:4245-4254.

[25] Liu, B., Zhao, H., Poon, M. C., et al. Abnormality of CD4(+)CD25(+) regulatory T cells in idiopathic thrombocytopenic purpura. *Eur. J. Haematol.* 2007; 78(2):139-143.

[26] Olsson, B., Andersson, P., Jernas, M., et al. T-cell-mediated cytotoxicity toward platelets in chronic idiopathic thrombocytopenic purpura. *Nat. Med.* 2003; 9:1123–1124.

[27] Houwerzijl, E. J., Blom, N. R., van der Want, J. J. L., et al. Ultrastructural study shows morphological features of apoptosis and para-apoptosis in megakaryocytes from patients with idiopathic thrombocytopenic purpura. *Blood* 2004; 103:500–506.

[28] Cines, D. B., Bussel, J. B., Liebman, H. A., and Luning Prak, E. T. The ITP syndrome: pathogenic and clinical diversity. *Blood* 2009; 113:6511-6521.

[29] Stasi, R., Sarpatwari, A., Segal, J. B., Osborn, J., Evangelista, M. L., Cooper, N., Provan, D., Newland, A., Amadori, A., Bussel, J. B. Effects of eradication of *Helicobacter pylori* infection in patients with immune thrombocytopenic purpura: a systematic review. *Blood* 2009; 113:1231-1240.

[30] Bussone, G., Mouthon, L. Autoimmune manifestations in primary immune deficiencies. *Autoimmune. Rev.* 2009; 8(4):332-336.

[31] Provan, D., Stasi, R., Newland, A. C., Blanchette, V. S., Bolton-Maggs, P., Bussel, J. B., Chong, B. H., Cines, D. B., Gernsheimer, T. B., Godeau, B., Grainger, J., Greer, I., Hunt, B. J., Imbach, P. A., Lyons, G., McMillan, R., Rodeghiero, F., Sanz, M. A., Tarantino, M., Watson, S., Young, J., Kuter, D. J. International consensus report on the investigation and management of primary immune thrombocytopenia. *Blood* 2010; 115: 168-186.

[32] Rodeghiero, F., Michel, M., Gernsheimer, T., Ruggeri, M., Blanchette, V., Bussel, J. B., Cines, D. B., Cooper, N., Godeau, B., Greinacher, A., Imbach, Khellaf, M., Klaassen, R. J., Kühne, T., Liebman, H., Mazzucconi, M. G., Newland, A., Pabinger, I., Tosetto, A., Stasi, R. Standardization of bleeding assessment in immune thrombocytopenia: report from the International Working Group. *Blood* 2013; 121:2596-2606.

[33] Thompson, C. B., Jakubowski, J. A. The pathophysiology and clinical relevance of platelet heterogeneity. *Blood* 1988; 72(1):1-8.

[34] Greene, L. A., Chen, S., Seery, C., Imahiyerobo, A. M., Bussel, J. B. Beyond the platelet count: immature platelet fraction and thromboelastometry correlate with bleeding in patients with immune thrombocytopenia. *Br. J. Haematol.* 2014; May 5. doi: 10.1111/bjh.12929.

[35] Rodeghiero, F., Stasi, R., Gernsheimer, T., et al. Standardization of terminology, definitions and outcome criteria in immune thrombocytopenic purpura of adults and children: report from the international working group. *Blood* 2009; 113(11):2386-2393.

[36] Cheng, Y., Wong, R. S. M., Soo, O. Y., Chui, C. H., Lau, F. Y., Chan, N. P. H., Wong, W. S., Cheng, G. Initial Treatment of Immune Thrombocytopenic Purpura with High-Dose Dexamethasone. *N. Engl. J. Med.* 2003; 349:831-836.

[37] Mazzucconi, M. G., Fazi, P., Bernasconi, S., De Rossi, G., Leone, G., Gugliotta, L., Vianelli, N., Avvisati, G., Rodeghiero, F., Amendola, A., Baronci, C., Carbone, C., Quattrin, S., Fioritoni, G., D'Alfonso, G., Mandelli, F., and for the Gruppo Italiano Malattie EMatologiche dell'Adulto (GIMEMA) Thrombocytopenia Working Party Therapy with high-dose dexamethasone (HD-DXM) in previously untreated patients affected by idiopathic thrombocytopenic purpura: a GIMEMA experience. *Blood* 2007; 109:1401-1407.

[38] Bae, S. H., Ryoo, H. M., Lee, W. S., Joo, Y. D., Lee, K. H., Lee Je-Hwan, Lee Jung-Hee, Kim, H., Park, J. H., Kim, M. K., Hyun, M. S., Kim, H. J., Zang, D. Y. High Dose Dexamethasone Vs. Conventional Dose Prednisolone for Adults with Immune Thrombocytopenia: a Prospective Multicenter Phase III Trial. *Blood* (ASH Annual Meeting Abstracts), Nov. 2010; 116: 3687.

[39] Imbach, P., Barandum, S., D'Apuzzo, V., et al. High-dose intravenous gammaglobulin for idiopathic thrombocytopenic purpura in childhood. *Lancet* 1981; 1:1228.

[40] Cooper, N., Heddle, N. M., Haas, M., et al. Intravenous (IV) anti-D and IV immunoglobulin achieve acute platelet increases by different mechanisms: modulation

of cytokine and platelet responses to IV anti-D by FcγRIIa and FcγRIIIa polymorphisms. *Br. J. Haematol.* 2004; 124(4):511-518.

[41] Pawlotsky, J. M., Bouvier, M., Deforges, L., et al. Chronic hepatitis C after high dose intravenous immunoglobulin. *Transfus.* 1994; 34:86.

[42] Crow, A. R. and Lazarus, A. H. The mechanisms of action of intravenous immunoglobulin and polyclonal anti-d immunoglobulin in the amelioration of immune thrombocytopenic purpura: what do we really know? *Transfus. Med. Rev.* 2008; 22(2): 103–116.

[43] Despotovic, J., Lambert, M. P., Herman, J., et al. RhIG for the treatment of immune thrombocytopenia: consensus and controversy. *Transfusion* 2012; (5):1126-1136.

[44] Zaja, F., Baccarani, M., Mazza, P., et al. Dexamethasone plus rituximab yields higher sustained response rates than dexamethasone monotherapy in adults with primary immune thrombocytopenia. *Blood* 2010; 115(14):2755-2762.

[45] Gudbrandsdottir, S., Birgens, H. S., Frederiksen, H., Jensen, A. B., Jensen, M. K., Kjeldsen, L., Klausen, T. W., Larsen, H., Mourits-Andersen, H. T., Nielsen, C. H., Nielsen, O. J., Plesner, T., Pulczynski, S., Rasmussen, I. H., Ronnov-Jessen, D., Hasselbalch, H. C. Rituximab and dexamethasone vs dexamethasone monotherapy in newly diagnosed patients with primary immune thrombocytopenia. *Blood* 2013; 121: 1976-1981.

[46] Stasi, R., Del Poeta, G., Stipa, E., et al. Response to B-cell depleting therapy with rituximab reverts the abnormalities of T-cell subsets in patients with idiopathic thrombocytopenic purpura. *Blood* 2007; 110:2924–2930.

[47] Stasi, R., Cooper, N., Del Poeta, G., et al. Analysis of regulatory T-cell changes in patients with idiopathic thrombocytopenic purpura receiving B cell-depleting therapy with rituximab. *Blood* 2008; 112(8):1147–1150.

[48] Audia, S., Samson, M., Mahévas, M., Ferrand, C., Trad, M., Ciudad, M., Gautheron, A., Seaphanh, F., Leguy, V., Berthier, S., Salles, B., Martin, L., Lorcerie, B., Ortega-Deballon, P., Facy, O., Caillot, D., Soudry-Faure, A., Michel, M., Godeau, B., Larmonier, N., Saas, P., Janikashvili, N., Bonnotte, B. Preferential splenic $CD8^+$ T-cell activation in rituximab-nonresponder patients with immune thrombocytopenia. *Blood* 2013; 122:2477-2486.

[49] Mahevas, M., Patin, P., Huetz, F., et al. B cell depletion in immune thrombocytopenia reveals splenic long-lived plasma cells. *J. Clin. Invest.* 2013; 123(1):432–442.

[50] Auger, S., Duny, Y., Rossi, J. F., Quittet, P. Rituximab before splenectomy in adults with primary idiopathic thrombocytopenic purpura: a meta-analysis. *British Journal of Haematology* 2012;158:386-398.

[51] Hasan, A., Michel, M., Patel, V., Stasi, R., Cunningham-Rundles, S., Leonard, J. P., Bussel, J. Repeated courses of rituximab in chronic ITP: three different regimens. *Am. J. Hematol.* 2009; 84:661-665.

[52] Lee, C. S., Imahiyerobo, A., Thompson, M., Karaev, M. I., Ghanima, W., Bussel, J. B. Rituximab Combined With Three Cycles Of High Dose Dexamethasone Provides a Long Term Response Rate Similar To That Of Splenectomy In Patients With Immune Thrombocytopenia (ITP) Of Duration Less Than 2 Years. *Blood* 2013; 122:2310.

[53] Mahler, M., Hasan, A., Bussel, J. B. Rituximab Maintenance Treatment In Immune Mediated Thrombocytopenia (ITP) Including Evans Syndrome. *Blood.* (ASH Annual Meeting Abstracts), Nov. 2010; 116: 2523.

[54] Zaja, F., Vianelli, N., Volpetti, S., et al. Low-dose rituximab in adult patients with primary immune thrombocytopenia. *European Journal of Haematology* 2010; 85:329-334.

[55] Niitsu, N., Hagiwara, Y., Tanae, K., Kohri, M., Takahashi, N. Prospective Analysis of Hepatitis B Virus Reactivation in Patients With Diffuse Large B-Cell Lymphoma After Rituximab Combination Chemotherapy. *J. Clin. Oncol.* 2010; 28(34):5097-5100.

[56] Carson, K. R., Evens, A. M., Richey, E. A., Habermann, T. M., Focosi, D., Seymour, J. F., Laubach, J., Bawn, S. D., Gordon, L. I., Winter, J. N., Furman, R. R., Vose, J. M., Zelenetz, A. D., Mamtani, R., Raisch, D. W., Dorshimer, G. W., Rosen, S. T., Muro, K., Gottardi-Littell, N. R., Talley, R. L., Sartor, O., Green, D., Major, E. O., Bennett, C. L. Progressive multifocal leukoencephalopathy after rituximab therapy in HIV-negative patients: a report of 57 cases from the Research on Adverse Drug Events and Reports project. *Blood* 2009; 113:4834-4840.

[57] Schwartz, J., Leber, M. D., Gillis, S., Eldor, A., Giunta, A., Bussel, J. B. Long term follow up after splenectomy performed for immune thrombocytopenic purpura. (ITP) *Am. J. Hematol.* 2003; 72(2)94-98.

[58] Budzynski, A., Bobrzynski, A., Sacha, T., Skotnicki, A. Laparoscopic removal of retroperitoneal accessory spleen in patients with relapsing idiopathic thrombocytopenic purpura 30 years after classical splenectomy. *Surg. Endosc.* 2002; 16(11):1636.

[59] Provan, D. International consensus report on the investigation and management of primary immune thrombocytopenia. *Blood* 2010;115(2)168-186.

[60] Boyle, S., White, R., Brunson, A., Wun, T. Splenectomy and incidence of venous thromboembolism and sepsis in patients with immune thrombocytopenia. *Blood* 2013; 121(23) 4782-4790.

[61] Alexakis, N., Dardamanis, D., Albanopoulos, K., et al. Incidence, risk factors, and outcome of portal thrombosis after laparoscopic-assisted splenectomy in β-thalassemia patients: a prospective exploratory study. *J. Laparoendosc. Adv. Surg. Tech. A.* 2013; 23(2):123-128.

[62] Crary, S., Buchanan, G. Vascular complications after splenectomy for hematologic disorders. *Blood* 2009;114(14)2861-2868.

[63] Nazi, I., Kelton, J. G., Larché, M., Snider, D. P., Heddle, N. M., Crowther, M. A., Cook, R. J., Tinmouth, A. T., Mangel, J., Arnold, D. M. The effect of rituximab on vaccine responses in patients with immune thrombocytopenia. *Blood* 2013; 122(11) 1946-1953.

[64] Thomsen, R. W., Schoonen, W. M., Farkas, D. K., et al. Risk of hospital contact with infections in patients with splenectomy: a population based cohort study. *Ann. Intern. Med.* 2009; 151(8):546-555.

[65] Keidar, A., Feldman, M., Szold, A. Analysis of outcome of laparoscopic splenectomy for idiopathic thrombocytopenic purpura by platelet count. *Am. J. Hematol.* 2005; 80 (2)95-100.

[66] Quah, C., Ayiomamitis, G. D., Shah, A., Ammori, B. J., Computer thomography to detect accessory spleens before laparoscopic splenectomy: is it necessary? *Surg. Endosc.* 2011; 25(1):261-265.

[67] Nakaseko, C., Togasaki, E., Shimizu, N., Sakaida, E. Partial Splenic Embolization For The Treatment Of Steroid-Resistant Chronic Idiopathic Thrombocytopenic Purpura. *Blood* 2013; 122(21):3543.

[68] Kuter, D. J. Romiplostim. *Cancer Treat. Res.* 2011; 157:267-288.

[69] Bussel, J. B., Pinheiro, M. P. Eltrombopag. *Cancer Treat. Res.* 2011; 157: 289-303.

[70] Cheng, G., Saleh, M. N., Marcher, C., et al. Eltrombopag for management of chronic immune thrombocytopenia (RAISE): a 6-month, randomised, phase 3 study. *The Lancet* 2011; 377(29):393-402.

[71] Saleh, M. N., Bussel, J. B., Cheng, G., et al. Safety and efficacy of eltrombopag for treatment of chronic immune thrombocytopenia: results of the long term, open-label EXTEND study. *Blood* 2013; 121(3):537-545.

[72] Bussel, J. B., Saleh, M. N., Wong, S. M,. et al. Update on the saftery and efficacy of EXTENDed treatment with Eltrombopag (EPAG) in adults with chronic immune thrombocytopenia (ITP). *Blood* 2013; 122(15):2315.

[73] Kuter, D. J., Phil, D., Rummel, M., et al. Romiplostin or Standard of Care in Patients with Immune Thrombocytopenia. *N. Engl. J. Med.* 2010;363(20):1889-1899.

[74] Janssens, A., Tarantiono, M., Bird, R., et al. Final Results from an International , Multi-Center, Single-Arm study evaluating the Safety and Efficay of Romiplostin in adults with Immune Thrombocytopenia (ITP) *Blood* 2011; 118:3279.

[75] Bussel, J. B., Wang, X., Eisen, M. Case Studies of Remission In Adults With Immune Thrombocytopenia (ITP) Following Cessation of Treatment With The TPO Receptor Agonist Romiplostim. *Blood* 2013; 122:328.

[76] Ghadaki, B. 1., Nazi, I., Kelton, J. G., Arnold, D. M. Sustained remissions of immune thrombocytopenia associated with the use of thrombopoietin receptor agonists. *Transfusion* 2013; 53(11):2807-2812.

[77] Mahévas, M., Fain, O., Ebbo, M., Khellaf, M., Limal, N., Schleinitz, N., Haioun, C., Bierling, P., Godeau, B., Michel, M. IV Prolonged Remission After TPO-Receptor Agonist Discontinuation In Adults With Chronic ITP. Results Of a French Observational Study. *Blood* 2013; 122:327.

[78] Gómez-Almaguer, D., Herrera-Rojas, M. A., Jaime-Pérez, J. C., Gómez-De León, A., Cantú-Rodríguez, O. G., Gutiérrez-Aguirre, C. H., Tarín-Arzaga, L., Hernández-Reyes, J., Ruiz-Arguelles, G. J. Eltrombopag and high-dose dexamethasone as frontline treatment for newly diagnosed immune thrombocytopenia in adults. *Blood* 2014; May 6. [Epub. ahead of print].

[79] Arumugaswamy, A., He, S., Quach, H., Brotchie, J., Grigg, A. Thrombopoietin receptor agonists in immune thrombocytopenia of less than 6 month duration. *Internal Medicine Journal* 2014; (44):519.

[80] McMillan, R., Durette, C. Long-term outcomes in adults with chronic ITP after splenectomy failure. *Blood* 2004;104(4):956-960.

[81] Boruchov, D. M., Gururangan, S., Driscoll, M. C., Bussel, J. B. Multiagent induction and maintenance therapy for patients with refractory immune thrombocytopenic purpura (ITP.) *Blood* 2007; 110:3526-3531.

[82] Arnold, D. M., Nazi, I., Santos, A., Chan, H., Heddle, N. M., Warkentin, T. E., Kelton, J. G. Combination immunosuppressant therapy for patients with chronic refractory immune thrombocytopenic purpura. *Blood* 2010; 115:29-31.

[83] Gudbrandsdottir, S., Leven, E., Imahiyerobo, A., Lee, S., Bussel, J. B. Cyclosporine-Romiplostim-IVIG Combination Therapy in Patients with Severe Immune Thrombocytopenia (ITP). *Blood* 2013; 122:1085.

[84] Rodeghiero, F., Ruggeri, M. Is splenectomy still the gold standard for the treatment of chronic ITP? *Am. J. Hematol.* 2008; 83(2):91.

[85] Bussel, J. B., Kuter, D. J., Pullarkat, V., Lyons, R. M., Guo, M., Nichol, J. L. Safety and efficacy of long-term treatment with romiplostim in thrombocytopenic patients with chronic ITP. *Blood* 2009; 113(10):2161-2171.

[86] Webert, K. E., Mittal, R., Sigouin, C., Heddle, N. M., Kelton, J. G. A retrospective 11-year analysis of obstetric patients with idiopathic thrombocytopenic purpura. *Blood* 2003; 102(13):4306-4311.

[87] Samuels, P., Bussel, J. B., Braitman, L. E., et al. Estimation of the risk of thrombocytopenia in the offspring of pregnant women with presumed immune thrombocytopenic purpura. *N. Engl. J. Med.* 1990; 323(4):229-235.

[88] Letsky, E. A., Greaves, M. Guidelines on the investigation and management of thrombocytopenia in pregnancy and neonatal alloimmune thrombocytopenia. Maternal and Neonatal Haemostasis Working Party of the Haemostasis and Thrombosis Task Force of the British Society for Haematology. *Br. J. Haematol.* 1996; 95(1):21-26.

[89] Park-Wyllie, L., Mazzotta, P., Pastuszak, A., et al. Birth defects after maternal exposure to corticosteroids: prospective cohort study and meta-analysis of epidemiological studies. *Teratology* 2000; 62(6):385-392.

[90] Roberts, D., Dalziel, S. Antenatal corticosteroids for accelerating fetal lung maturation for women at risk of preterm birth. *Cochrane Database Syst. Rev.* 2006; 19(3):CD0044 54 Review.

[91] Webert, K. E., Mittal, R., Sigouin, C., Heddle, N. M., Kelton, J. G. A retrospective 11-year analysis of obstetric patients with idiopathic thrombocytopenic purpura. *Blood* 2003; 102(13):4306-4311.

[92] Burrows, R., Kelton, J. G. Fetal thrombocytopenia and its relation to maternal thrombocytopenia. *N. Engl. J. Med.* 1993; 329(20):1463–1466.

[93] Gernssheimer, T. Thrombocytopenia in pregnancy: is this immune thrombocytopenia or …? *American Society of Hematology Education Book* 2012; 198-202.

[94] Felbinger, T. W., Posner, M., Eltzschig, H. K., Kodali, B. S. Laparoscopic splenectomy in a pregnant patient with immune thrombocytopenic purpura. *Int. J. Obstet. Anesth.* 2007; 16(3):281-283.

[95] Ghanima, W., Godeau, B., Cines, D. B., Bussel, J. B. How I treat immune thrombocytopenia: the choice between splenectomy or a medical therapy as a second-line treatment. *Blood* 2012; 120:960-969.

[96] Gernsheimer, T., James, A. H., Stasi, R. How I treat thrombocytopenia in pregnancy. *Blood* 2013; 121(1): 38-47.

[97] Salama, A., Kiesewetter, H., Kalus, U., Movassaghi, K., Meyer, O. Massive platelet transfusion is a rapidly effective emergency treatment in patients with refractory autoimmune thrombocytopenia. *Thromb. Haemost.* 2008; 100(5):762-765.

[98] Boruchov, D. M., Gururangan, S., Driscoll, M. C., Bussel, J. B. Multiagent induction and maintenance therapy for patients with refractory immune thrombocytopenic purpura (ITP). *Blood* 2007; 110(10):3526-3531.

[99] Monroe, D. M., Hoffman, M., Oliver, J. A., Roberts, H. R. Platelet activity of high-dose factor VIIa is independent of tissue factor. *Br. J. Haematol.* 1997; 99(3):542–547.

[100] Young, G., Wicklund, B., Neff, P., et al. Off-label use of rFVIIa in children with excessive bleeding: a consecutive study of 153 off-label uses in 139 children. *Pediatr. Blood Cancer* 2009; 53(2):179–183.

In: Thrombocytopenia
Editor: Mckenzie G. Bell

ISBN: 978-1-63321-713-3

Chapter 2

The Approach to Thrombocytopenia in the Hospital Setting: A Primer for the General Internist

Debra A. Ferman, MD[1,*], Gita Lisker, MD[2,†], Alida Podrumar, MD[1,‡] and Alan S. Multz, MD[1,§]
[1]Nassau University Medical Center, East Meadow, NY, US
[2]North Shore Long Island Jewish Health System, New Hyde Park, NY, US

Abstract

Thrombocytopenia in the hospital setting is a common platelet related condition seen by clinicians in all disciplines. It may be the result of something acquired during that hospitalization or in the recent past or in some circumstances even after a recent hospitalization, or it can be result of a congenitally acquired disorder. In this chapter, we will discuss the following topics related to this disease: how infections and medications impact this disorder; the impact of some common medical conditions that predate a hospitalization and how these diseases may impact upon a patient with thrombocytopenia; the causes of severe thrombocytopenia as defined as a platelet count of less than 10,000/mm^3 and thrombocytopenia as it relates to pregnancy. We will discuss various aspects of these issues including the epidemiology, the definition of the problem, clinical presentation, diagnosis including laboratory evaluation and the differential diagnosis, the underlying pathophysiology as we understand I and, treatment options. At

* Debra A. Ferman, MD. Nassau University Medical Center, 2201 Hempstead Turnpike, East Meadow, NY 11554. (P): 516-572-6501, (f): 516-572-5609, e-mail: dferman@numc.edu, fermanator@optonline.net.
† Gita Lisker, MD. North Shore Long Island Jewish Health System, 410 Lakeville Road, Suite 107, New Hyde Park, NY 11040. (P) 516-465-5433, e-mail: Glisker2@nshs.edu, gitalisker@yahoo.com.
‡ Alida Podrumar, MD. Nassau University Medical Center, 2201 Hempstead Turnpike, East Meadow, NY 11554. (P): 516-572-6501, (f): 516-572-5609, e-mail: apodruma@numc.edu, alida70@hotmail.com.
§ Corresponding author: Alan S. Multz, MD. Nassau University Medical Center, 2201 Hempstead Turnpike, East Meadow, NY 11554. (P): 516-572-6501, (f): 516-572-5609, e-mail: amultz@numc.edu, multzman@optonline.net.

the conclusion of reading this chapter, the clinician should have a greater understanding of this spectrum of this problem.

Keywords: Thrombocytopenia, pregnancy

Introduction

The approach to thrombocytopenia in the hospital setting should be systematic and methodical. Most of the time, the etiology is unclear and one must make the best educated guess. In the ICU and surgical settings, at times one must choose between various clinical outcomes, as to which one would be worse for the patient. Is it worse to clot or worse to bleed? This decision should be made with the patient's involvement and in consultation with the primary surgeon or primary physician caring for the patient.

A good clinician works as a detective, using the tools of history and physical examination, with support of lab values and peripheral smear to arrive at a diagnosis. Ninety percent of the time, a diagnosis in adults may be made simply by taking a proper history. It is important to take the time to contact the patient's primary care physician and obtain prior platelet count values. A baseline low platelet count would change the top choices in the differential diagnosis in the hospitalized patient. If the thrombocytopenia developed during the hospitalization, the culprit is usually something acquired.

For example, one must consider exposure to the cardiac bypass pump during heart surgery and its relation to the drop in platelet count. Usually an acquired thrombocytopenia in the hospital setting is due to "bugs or drugs." Does the patient have an underlying condition causing disseminated intravascular coagulation (DIC)? Did the patient receive a blood transfusion 7 to 10 days prior to the drop in platelet count? These are all important questions that need to be asked.

To evaluate thrombocytopenia, one should make a diagram of the platelet count trend with dates, and then make note of where new medications were added and old ones were discontinued, including dates of surgery such as cardiac bypass and vascular surgery, as well as procedures such as cardiac catheterization. One should also document the exposure to various medications, including antibiotics, heparin, and warfarin. It is important to assess the timing of the platelet count drop in relation to medication exposures. This diagram helps one visualize the patient's hospital course in relation to his or her platelet count. The clinician's duty is to always assess the patient's risk for heparin induced thrombocytopenia, because missing this diagnosis could prove disastrous for the patient.

Physical examination may support your diagnosis. In the critical care setting, it is important to note all locations of active bleeding, including wound and drainage sites, central venous catheter and arterial line insertion sites, tracheostomy tube, nasogastric tube, Foley catheter, rectal tube, and IV locks. It is important to examine the skin for ecchymosis, purpura, petechiae and other signs of bleeding.

An extremity exam is also important, with assessment of the presence or absence of dorsalis pedis and posterior tibial pulses, gangrene, and edema. Blood blisters or wet purpura in the mouth often are predictive for risk of spontaneous bleeding in thrombocytopenia patients. Assessment for lymphadenopathy and hepatosplenomegaly may point towards a preexisting illness as a cause for the thrombocytopenia. When considering the diagnosis of lymphoma or leukemia, a testicular exam should be performed.

In the hospital setting, various lab values could be helpful. It is imperative to obtain a basic CBC with differential, INR, aPTT, fibrinogen, and D-dimer.

Based on the detective work, the lab testing then broadens. The level of thrombocytopenia may provide a clue to potential diagnosis. Usually a platelet count of less than 10,000/mm^3 points to only a few etiologies: a drug induced thrombocytopenia (including GPIIb/IIIa inhibitors), ITP, post-transfusion purpura, and at times DIC. A bone marrow biopsy is usually not very helpful in assessing acquired thrombocytopenia in the hospital setting, but may be extremely valuable in the evaluation of a pre-existing thrombocytopenia. An abdominal sonogram may reveal splenomegaly and show evidence of liver disease. In most cases, this may be picked up during a proper physical examination. The peripheral smear usually remains within the purview of the consulting hematologist. To be able to make a diagnosis simply on peripheral smear can be rewarding.

A case in point was the peripheral smear of a patient in the cardiothoracic intensive care unit that had recently undergone heart surgery, and had post-operative hypotension without fever. The peripheral smear showed Dohle bodies and toxic granulation, which pointed to a clinical picture that was consistent with sepsis. Antibiotics were recommended.

The goal of this chapter is to help guide the clinician through the world of thrombocytopenia in the hospital setting and provide a comprehensive review of common causes.

Part 1: Acquired Thrombocytopenia in the Hospital Setting: Bugs or Drugs

- Infection
- Drugs Induced Thrombocytopenia
    - Medications
    - Special cases – individual drugs
    - Oxaliplatin induced thrombocytopenia
    - Heparin induced thrombocytopenia (HIT)
    - Glycoprotein IIb/IIIa antagonists (see part 3)
- Post-transfusion purpura
- Disseminated intravascular coagulation (DIC)
- Dilutional thrombocytopenia
- Mechanical intravascular devices –cardiac bypass pump, intra-aortic balloon pump

Introduction

When one tackles the problem of thrombocytopenia in the hospital setting, it is important to note the time course. Part 1 focuses on problems associated with new onset thrombocytopenia during the hospital stay. If the patient came in with a normal count and then it dropped, it is most certainly the result of an infection, medication, medical intervention, or a medical device. The clinical scenario is critical to figure out the cause and the timeliness of treatment. If there is an abrupt drop in platelet count with recent surgery, one can think of post-transfusion purpura, a drug induced thrombocytopenia, or HIT [1]. Intensive Care Unit (ICU) thrombocytopenia is another term for thrombocytopenia in the critically ill. The development of thrombocytopenia in the ICU is a predictor for mortality [2]. Infection is a common cause, as well as many other reasons that will be discussed in this chapter.

Infection

The diagnosis and clinical presentation of thrombocytopenia can be related to many infections, including bacterial, viral, fungal and parasitic. Infective endocarditis commonly has a low platelet count and the diagnosis is made by obtaining blood cultures. In endocarditis, the platelet count could be low or normal in number. Sepsis may cause a mild thrombocytopenia of around 50,000/mm^3 [3]. When the platelet count is less than 50,000/mm^3, there could be concomitant disseminated intravascular coagulation (DIC) [3]. Malaria and Epstein Barr (EBV) viral infection may also cause an acute thrombocytopenia [3]. The peripheral smear findings in severe bacterial infection can be as follows: one may see increased bands, Dohle bodies, neutrophil vacuoles or presence of toxic granulation of the neutrophils [4].

The pathophysiology of infection related thrombocytopenia is proposed as follows. Platelets are a step in the host defense against bacteria [5]. Certain bacteria induce platelet activation by binding to PF4 and being recognized by circulating IgG [5]. In infective endocarditis, platelet activation may contribute to the build-up of platelets, fibrin, and bacteria on the heart valves [6]. Embolization of these clots may cause small cerebral infarcts [6].

In bacteremia there may be enhanced clearance of immune complex-coated platelets, decreased platelet production, and increased splenic sequestration [2]. Viral infections may affect megakaryocytes and suppress platelet production [2]. Sepsis-associated disseminated coagulopathy may occur when blood coagulation factors are consumed by microvascular thrombosis [6].

The treatment of infection related thrombocytopenia is to use appropriate antimicrobials to treat the underlying infectious cause.

Drug Induced Thrombocytopenia

Immune cytopenias can develop due to many drugs, including heparin, abciximab, quinine, quinidine, penicillin, ranitidine, rifampicin, and vancomycin [7]. The epidemiology of drug induced thrombocytopenias is that it can occur at any age and in any sex [8]. There are no known predisposing genetic or environmental factors [8]. Only a small percentage of patients develop this side effect, despite treating large numbers of patients [8]. The incidence may be higher in hospitalized patients and the elderly [8].

The diagnosis is best made by demonstrating an antibody in the serum that reacts to normal platelets in the presence of drug [9]. This is rarely done in clinical practice. Testing for drug induced antibodies is not widely available [8].

In addition, a patient can have a history typical for drug induced thrombocytopenia, but antibody tests may be negative because a drug metabolite is responsible [8]. The diagnosis of drug induced thrombocytopenia is often missed because patients are ill and have many other reasons for thrombocytopenia including infection, bypass surgery, and acute illness [8]. One should suspect the diagnosis in a patient with acute thrombocytopenia of unknown cause and it should be noted that the thrombocytopenia can be transient [8]. Sometimes patients are treated for immune thrombocytopenia until the drug has been identified [8]. It is very important to take a careful medication history, including herbal preparations [8].

The most common drugs classes to cause thrombocytopenia are heparins, chemotherapy agents, immunosuppressants, diuretics, antimicrobials, sedative agents, anticonvulsants, analgesics and platelet inhibiting agents. More extensive lists are available on the internet (http://moon.ouhsc.edu/jgeorge/DITP.html). Keep in mind that other drugs may also cause low platelet counts, but at much lower rates.

The clinical presentation of drug induced thrombocytopenia is typically five to seven days of exposure to a drug when giving a drug for the first time [8]. The usual time course for thrombocytopenia may be a week or a longer period for patients taking the drug intermittently [8]. Some patients develop a thrombocytopenia within 1 to 2 days of a first exposure to a drug [8]. They can have an associated syndrome with systemic symptoms of lightheadedness, fever, nausea, vomiting, and chills [8]. At this point, the platelet count is usually less than $20{,}000/mm^3$, and patients can develop epistaxis, gum bleeding, gastrointestinal bleeding, and purpura.

The peripheral smear findings in drug induced thrombocytopenia can be similar to those seen in ITP, accompanied by a low platelet count. One might also find the presence of moderately enlarged platelets [4].

The pathophysiology of drug induced thrombocytopenia is that exposure to the drug leads to the destruction of platelets by drug induced antibodies [8]. There are six mechanisms, classified as hapten-dependent antibody (penicillin), quinine-type drug (quinine, sulfonamides, NSAIDs), fiban-type drug (Tiroban, eptifibatide), drug specific antibody (Abciximab), autoantibody (gold salts, procainamide), and immune complex (heparins) [8]. Drug induced autoantibodies occur in the absence of a sensitizing agent [8]. Drugs that may cause autoantibody formation include procainamide, sulfonamide antibiotics, interferons alfa and beta.

The treatment of drug-induced immune thrombocytopenia is to discontinue the drug. Usually symptoms resolve in 2 days and the platelet count returns to normal within a week [8]. At times, it is unclear which drug is the offending agent. In this situation it is prudent to stop all medications [8]. When the diagnosis initially is uncertain, corticosteroids are given but should be tapered quickly once the culprit for the thrombocytopenia is determined. It has not been proven if corticosteroids are helpful [8]. IVIG and plasma exchange have been used in the acutely ill, but it is unclear if there is any benefit [8].

Once a patient has been diagnosed as having drug induced thrombocytopenia, this side effect persists and the patient should be told they have an allergy. The patient should be counseled to avoid the medication [8]. Drug induced antibodies are specific for certain drugs [8]. If the patient were to need a pharmacologic equivalent it could be tried, even if the drugs have similar structures [8].

Special Cases - Individual Drugs

Drug induced TTP occurs in 1/2500 patients receiving ticlopidine [8]. The incidence is less common with clopidogrel. With clopidogrel, the signs and symptoms start after 1-2 weeks of treatment [8].

Monoclonal antibodies like Rituximab (anti-CD 20 antibody) and infliximab (anti-tumor necrosis factor-alpha antibody) have also been shown to cause thrombocytopenia. The clinical presentation in this case is usually a self-limited thrombocytopenia [8].

In patients receiving valproic acid and linezolid, the clinical presentation in about thirty percent of patients receiving long-term treatment has been a low grade thrombocytopenia [8]. Usually the platelet count is not low enough to require treatment. The mechanism of the thrombocytopenia in this case may not be immune [8].

Oxaliplatin Induced Thrombocytopenia

Oxaliplatin (a platinum compound used in the treatment of colon cancer and other GI malignancies) induced immune thrombocytopenia is worth discussing. It presents clinically as an acute drop in platelet count after exposure, usually 1-3 days. It can occur after multiple exposures to the drug. The mechanism may be drug-induced rather than from suppressed hematopoiesis, which usually takes 7-10 days after exposure to cause a drop in platelet count. Hypersensitivity reactions to oxaliplatin occur 15% of the time [10]. They are more common in females but may occur in men [9]. Usually patients had several treatments of oxaliplatin in the past with no reaction [10]. A diagnosis of oxaliplatin induced immune thrombocytopenia is made after a hypersensitivity reaction occurs in a treated patient. At that time, it is important to check a CBC with differential, review the smear, order a direct antiglobulin test, a reticulocyte count, an LDH, and a haptoglobin [9]. Lab studies used to help diagnose hemolysis are recommended to ensure there is no drug-induced hemolytic uremic syndrome (HUS) [9]. The clinical presentation is as follows: the patient suffers an acute hypersensitivity reaction during or after the oxaliplatin infusion [10]. During the infusion there could be rigors, pyrexia, nausea, vomiting, fever, tachycardia, or dyspnea [10]. The platelet count drops immediately and there could also be hemolysis in these patients [10]. The patient may have symptomatic bleeding including gingival bleeding, epistaxis, petechiae, bruising, tongue hematoma, and a low platelet count [9, 10]. Most patients with Evans syndrome, immune hemolysis and immune thrombocytopenia, develop back pain during the oxaliplatin infusion [9]. The peripheral smear findings in oxaliplatin induced immune thrombocytopenia include decreased platelets, normal morphology and no schistocytes [9].

The pathophysiology here is an example of hematologic toxicity when a patient has an acute reaction to drug [10]. Platelet destruction occurs by oxaliplatin dependent IgG antibodies specific for the platelet glycoprotein IIb/IIIa [9, 10]. From oxaliplatin adsorption, there is the development of autoantibodies to blood cells and there is release of proinflammatory molecules IL-6 and TNF alpha [10]. This could potentially explain the infusion reaction. The treatment for a hypersensitivity reaction to oxaliplatin is to first stop the oxaliplatin and then treat with steroids and antihistamines [9].

It is important to check CBC and monitor the patient for bleeding, as platelets drop within 24 hours of the infusion [9]. Platelet transfusion is given as needed. It is uncertain if corticosteroids are helpful [9]. The recovery of the platelet count usually occurs within a week or two after stopping oxaliplatin [9, 10]. The patient should be notified of an allergy to oxaliplatin and never take the drug again [9].

Heparin Induced Thrombocytopenia (HIT)

HIT is a prothrombotic drug reaction [11]. We know that thrombocytopenia is common in hospitalized patients and HIT is only a small subset [12]. Keeping that in mind, HÎT is the most common drug reaction involving blood cells [13]. It can be further characterized as HIT without thrombosis (HIT) or HIT with thrombosis (HITT).

HIT incidence is 0.2% to 5% of all adults treated with heparin [14]. Unfractionated heparin (UFH) exposure poses a greater risk to develop HIT compared to low molecular weight heparin (LMWH) [14]. One study showed that being female and surgical patients had a higher incidence [14]. HIT was also more common in trauma patients [14]. As well, certain surgeries had an increased risk of HIT, including cardiopulmonary bypass [14]. Five percent of patients who were treated with UFH thromboprophylaxis after major orthopedic surgery developed HIT [14].

HIT is rare in patients under the age of 40 [14]. It is uncommon, less than 0.1% in pregnant patients [14]. HIT occurs less than 1% of the time in critically ill patients and hemodialysis patients [14]. However, the incidence of thrombocytopenia in the ICU could be as high as 50% [14].

The diagnosis of HIT is based on clinical suspicion, pretest probability, and lab testing [11]. The diagnosis requires a consistent clinical picture and the detection of platelet activating antibodies [12]. To diagnose HIT based on lab testing one must order the IgG specific ELISA immunoassay (EIA) and the serotonin release assay (SRA) test [12].

The 4Ts scoring system can be used as a guide to assessing the likelihood of HIT. A low probability score is a good way to exclude HIT and an intermediate or high probability score requires further investigation [11]. The negative predictive value of a low probability score was 0.998 regardless of the prevalence of HIT in a patient population [11]. The positive predictive value of a high score was 0.64 and an intermediate score was 0.14 [11].

Lab assays include immunoassays which are common to have false positive results [11]. The solid-phase ELISA immunoassay can be explained as follows: "PF4/polyanion or PF4/ heparin complexes are coated onto microtiter plate wells and patient serum is added. If serum contains IgG, IgA, or IgM antibodies, then it will bind to the complex and can be detected by addition of secondary anti-isotype antibodies." [14] The PF4 dependent EIA detects HIT irrelevant antibodies [12]. This test has a low positive predictive value but a highly negative predictive value [14]. A negative EIA rules out HIT [12]. False positives may occur due to antiphospholipid antibodies [14]. There is also an IgG-specific ELISA test, since it is thought that the IgG antibodies are the main cause for clinical HIT [14]. Limiting the test to only IgG antibodies increases the specificity but decreases the sensitivity [14]. Some labs add another step to the test, where high dose heparin is added and if this inhibits the positive ELISA by more than 50%, this confirms the presence of heparin-dependent antibodies [14].

There also are functional lab assays for HIT which is not standardized [11]. There are washed platelet function assays such as the SRA, which has greater specificity, but in order to perform the test requires radioisotope and reactive donor platelets [11]. The results of this test never come back in a clinically useful time frame. The functional assays have a greater specificity but a lower sensitivity than the ELISA test [15]. The SRA discerns which heparin-induced antibodies are clinically relevant and should be ordered when an ELISA test is positive [12].

The following is a brief clinical description of the 4Ts scoring system. There are four categories: **T**hrombocytopenia, **T**iming, **T**hrombosis, and O**t**her. Each category is assigned a numerical score of 0, 1 or 2 adding up to a maximum score of 8. For thrombocytopenia, a drop below 20,000/mm^3 is not really consistent with HIT and gets zero points for that category. The degree of thrombocytopenia is important. For a patient with a baseline platelet count of 800,000/mm^3, a drop to 300,000/mm^3 would be more than a 50% decline and could be consistent with HIT [14]. One would get 2 points in that category. For timing of the platelet count drop with respect to heparin exposure, a score of 2 is given when the platelets drop within 5 to 10 days of exposure or less than 1 day if the patient was exposed to heparin within the past 30 days [11]. The presence of thrombosis increases the chance for HIT and one gets a score of 2 in that category. One must also consider whether other factors that cause thrombocytopenia are present. If definitely present, then one gets a score of 0. A score of 0 to 3 is low probability and one could feel comfortable that the diagnosis is not HIT and not even order the ELISA antibody test. Unfortunately, many cases in the hospital setting have a score in the moderate range of 4 to 5, thus leaving the clinical decision to the clinician. In these circumstances, the question remains, is it worse for the patient to bleed or clot? The scores for pretest probability are useful to exclude HIT [12]. Even with a high probability score of 6 to 8 on the nomogram, only 50% of patients have a positive SRA [12].

The level of optical density (OD) is a marker of antibody levels [12]. An OD of 0.5 means that there is less than a 5% probability for true HIT. An OD of 1.5 is 25%, OD of 2.5 is 95%, and OD of less than 0.4 is 0% probability for true HIT [12]. An OD greater than 2 has a greater than 90% probability of HIT [12]. At this level, an SRA usually is not needed.

At present, there is a problem of over diagnosis of HIT. Misdiagnosis of HIT may cause harm. The exposure of thrombocytopenic patients to alternative anticoagulants with no antidote can result in a 1% daily risk of major hemorrhage and the patient could also develop thrombosis from needlessly stopping heparin [11]. In addition, the direct thrombin inhibitors are very expensive. As such it is recommended to order the ELISA test and the platelet activation assay. If the pre-test probability for HIT is low, then do not order the test [12]. There is no need to order repeat HIT antibodies on subsequent days [12].

Despite thrombocytopenia, HIT is a prothrombotic state (13). The clinical presentation of HIT may be as thrombocytopenia with or without thrombosis during or after heparin treatment [15]. Typical HIT can present with either or both venous or arterial thromboembolism [16]. Untreated HIT may result in new thromboses, amputation, and death. In post cardiac surgery patients with HIT, arterial thrombi predominate although DVT and PE also are common [17]. Upper limb DVT also may occur especially in the setting of a central venous catheter [17].

The physical exam is notable for the absence of petechiae and bleeding [14]. Cyanosis and gangrene of the digits with preserved pulses may also occur [14]. Thrombosis could occur anywhere, including cerebral sinuses, adrenal veins with hemorrhage and failure, and graft occlusion [14]. Skin necrosis at a subcutaneous injection site and anaphylaxis with intravenous heparin boluses can rarely occur [14]. There have been reports of hypotension and dyspnea in patients with HIT upon reexposure to heparin [16].

Delayed HIT is a distinct syndrome that develops several days after stopping heparin [13]. Think of the diagnosis when a recently hospitalized patient presents with thrombosis [16]. Even a slightly low platelet count could be a clue, and early treatment with an alternative anticoagulant is recommended [16]. Usually such patients had a prior benign hospital course which included exposure to heparin. Delayed HIT may occur from 9 to 40 days later, with a median of 14 days [16].

Rarely there has been severe HIT with a platelet count nadir of less than 20,000 and this is due to a concomitant coagulopathy [12].

The peripheral smear findings in HIT may be normal with the platelet count usually being low as described above.

The pathophysiology of HIT is detailed and well known. There are platelet activating IgG antibodies against multi-molecular complexes of Platelet Factor 4 (PF4) and heparin or platelet factor 4 (PF4) and polyanion complexes [11, 12]. These antibodies are already detectable at the beginning of the platelet count decline, and include IgG, IgA, and IgM [12]. Only a small percentage of anti-PF4/Heparin antibodies are platelet activating [12]. Only IgG antibodies can activate the platelets and IgG specific EIA tests are now performed [12]. In general, anti-PF4 antibodies decrease within 90 days.

Platelet Factor 4 (PF4) is stored in the alpha granules of the platelet and is released upon activation of the platelet [13]. PF4 is positively charged and forms complexes with the polyanions of heparin [13]. PF4 complexed to heparin forms neoepitopes that are targeted by antibodies [13]. The fact that HIT antibodies develop in 5 days, suggests that patients have been pre-immunized against PF4/polyanion complexes, possibly during a prior infection with PF4 coated bacteria [13]. It is postulated that anti-PF4 heparin antibodies may be part of a bacterial host defense mechanism [13]. As mentioned in the "Infection" section, certain bacteria bind to PF4 and are recognized by antibodies [5].

The risk of developing anti-PF4/heparin antibodies is greater in the setting of trauma or inflammation [13]. Cardiopulmonary bypass (CPB) causes mechanical tissue damage, ischemia reperfusion injury, serum cytokines, and a strong inflammatory response [13].

A proposed mechanism for delayed HIT is that some anti-PF4/heparin antibodies are similar to autoantibodies which bind to PF4 on platelets in the absence of heparin [13]. For this reason, the syndrome develops after heparin is no longer administered [13].

The treatment of HIT can be started once there is significant suspicion for the diagnosis. If the 4Ts score is low probability, then one can safely exclude HIT and continue heparin without any lab testing [11]. Delayed recognition and treatment lead to poor patient outcomes [16].

In untreated HIT, in the first two days after stopping heparin the risk for thrombosis is 5-10% and the incidence of thrombosis at 30 days is 50% [14]. When HIT is suspected, it is important to order a lower extremity Doppler as well as to discontinue the heparin immediately including all line flushes [11]. Until lab results come back, the management is based on clinical judgement of the likelihood for HIT [12]. One should not treat the patient with oral Vitamin K antagonists such as warfarin until the platelet count has recovered [11]. Immediate treatment with a non-heparin anticoagulant is warranted [11, 14]. Any delays in treatment could result in a 5 to 10% daily risk of thrombosis, including amputation and death [11]. The decision of initiating direct thrombin inhibitor treatment must be individualized and assess the potential risks and benefits of each patient [11].

Argatroban is a direct thrombin inhibitor cleared by the liver [14]. It can be given at reduced doses in the setting of liver failure, heart failure, anasarca, and post-cardiac surgery [14]. With direct thrombin inhibitors, there is a 10-20% incidence of hemorrhage and there is no antidote if a bleeding complication occurs [14]. However, the half-life of Argatroban is relatively short, at 45 minutes.

Argatroban should be started immediately when the diagnosis is suspected. The direct thrombin inhibitor may be stopped after day 5, when the INR is therapeutic. With regard to

Argatroban titration, one keeps the aPTT 1.5 to 3 times the baseline aPTT value of the patient, not to exceed 100 seconds. Argatroban increases the INR and a therapeutic range usually is greater than 4. Complex algorithms exist for proper titration of the argatroban. Usually, what is needed is to aim for an INR of over 4.

Once the INR is over 4 while the aPTT is therapeutic, one stops the Argatroban and waits 6 hours. At 6 hours, an INR and an aPTT are repeated. If the aPTT is normal, this confirms that the Argatroban has been cleared from the system and then the INR is the true reading. At this point therapeutic would be an INR over 2.

Bivalirudin is a direct thrombin inhibitor used in the setting of percutaneous vascular procedures and is often used during cardiac catheterization specifically for HIT patients [14]. The half-life is even shorter at 25 minutes. Fondaparinux is an indirect inhibitor of Factor Xa which is approved for the prevention and treatment of venous thromboembolism [14]. There have been case series published of its use in HIT. It is administered subcutaneously and has a half-life of around 17 hours. Fondaparinux is likely effective treatment for HIT, but currently it is off label [12]. Fondaparinux has a role in use in patients with a history of HIT who need DVT prophylaxis and treatment.

If the diagnosis of HIT was delayed and the patient is already receiving warfarin, it is recommended to reverse the warfarin with vitamin K and stop the warfarin [14]. Warfarin use during acute HIT is a risk factor for limb gangrene [12]. Once the platelet count recovers to normal, one may start warfarin and overlap it with a direct thrombin inhibitor for 5 or more days [14]. The protein C deficiency that develops from warfarin could lead to hypercoagulability and for this reason overlap with a direct thrombin inhibitor is needed [14]. In addition, it is recommended to start at a low dose of 5 mg warfarin [14].

Warfarin therapy for approximately 3 months is recommended in the absence of thrombosis. In the presence of thrombosis, the length of treatment depends on the length of treatment recommended for the clot, anywhere from 3 to 6 months [14]. HIT is considered a transient risk factor for another VTE [14].

In the United States, once a patient is diagnosed as having HIT, it is recommended not to take heparin again. There are certain situations however, when heparin is unavoidable, including certain procedures. Preoperatively, one should obtain HIT ELISA antibody and serotonin release assay. If both tests are negative, the patient may receive heparin but only during the intraoperative or procedure setting, and heparin should be avoided pre and post operatively [14, 17]. Re-exposure to heparin in the perioperative setting is feasible if necessary and the risk for causing HIT again are low but not zero [18]. The CBC should be monitored closely and the patient should be counseled that there is a risk that HIT may develop again. Consultation with a hematologist should be considered.

In hemodialysis patients with a history of HIT, alternative flushing strategies including saline, citrate, and argatroban have been reported as well as long term warfarin use [14].

In HIT, one should avoid a platelet transfusion unless there is active bleeding, as it is known to worsen thrombosis [14]. It may be necessary to consider platelet transfusion however, if there is clinically significant bleeding or if there is a high bleeding risk present [14].

Post-Transfusion Purpura

The epidemiology of post-transfusion purpura is such that the incidence is 1 out of 200,000 transfusions [20].

It is more common in multiparous women who were sensitized during pregnancy [1, 4]. Patients may also be sensitized during prior transfusion (Christie). The diagnosis is made by detecting the antibody to a platelet allo-antigen [4]. Common alloantigen targets are human platelet antigens HPA-1a and HPA-5b [19].

Other alloantigen targets include HPA-3a, HPA-3b, and HPA-4a [20]. These alloantigens are located on the GPIIb/IIIa or GP1a/IIa complexes on platelets [20].

The clinical presentation is seen when a patient with a normal platelet count receives a transfusion of packed red cells (PRBC) and then 7 to 10 days later develops severe thrombocytopenia [20]. Post-transfusion purpura may occur within the time course of 5 to 15 days after a blood product, usually a red cell transfusion [4]. Patients are exposed to this platelet antigen in the transfused red cells [20].

The unique feature is that the donor platelets and the patient's own non allogeneic platelets are destroyed, thus causing a severe thrombocytopenia below 10,000/mm^3 [20]. The risk of intracerebral bleed is highest early in the course of illness [19]. Severe hemorrhage and postsurgical bleeding may also occur [20]. The peripheral smear finding in this disorder is usually the presence of large platelets [20].

The pathophysiology of post transfusion purpura is that the patient develops an alloantibody to a platelet antigen, usually anti-HPA-1a but other HPA antigens have been implicated [4]. The HPA-1a antibody reacts with the donor platelets, destroying them and the recipient's own platelets [1].

The treatment usually requires management decisions to be made before the antibody test result comes back. Platelet transfusions are recommended for patients with post-transfusion purpura and life threatening bleeding [19]. Ideally HPA-1a negative platelets are given [1]. A moderate increase in platelet count was seen with transfusion of HPA-1a/5b negative platelets [19]. A lack of response to platelet transfusion is associated with significant bleeding complications [20]. Treatment for this disorder is intravenous immunoglobulin (IVIG) given over 2 or 5 days [1, 19]. Glucocorticoids are also given [4]. Plasmapheresis is also a potential treatment option [1].

Disseminated Intravascular Coagulation (DIC)

The epidemiology is intimately related to the question one must ask, which is whether there is an underlying disorder associated with DIC [1]. Some conditions associated with DIC include sepsis, severe infection, trauma, pancreatitis, malignancy, vascular abnormalities and aneurysm, and severe liver failure [21]. The diagnosis of DIC is a dynamic diagnosis and usually one needs at least two points in time to assess the thrombocytopenia and coagulation tests. Lab values in DIC show a prolonged INR and aPTT, low fibrinogen, increased D-dimer, prolonged bleeding time, decreased platelet count, low activated protein C levels and elevated fibrin degradation products [1].

The clinical presentation of DIC is due to the fact that it is an acquired syndrome where there is intravascular activation of coagulation with loss of localization, arising from different causes [1]. To make the diagnosis of DIC, it is important to evaluate the pattern of bleeding, whether it is generalized or localized. In fulminant DIC, oozing occurs at vascular access sites and wounds, and there is profuse hemorrhage [1].

Symptoms of DIC include hemorrhage, and 5-10% can develop digital ischemia [1]. Widespread petechiae and mucosal bleeding may also be a sign of a platelet disorder [1]. At times, it is difficult to distinguish end stage liver disease from DIC [1].

The peripheral smear findings are important to recognize. These might include a microangiopathic smear with a low platelet count, occasional schistocytes (fragmented red cells) and possibly the presence of Burr cells [4].

The pathophysiology has been extensively studied. The mechanism of DIC originates in the microvasculature and causes organ dysfunction [1]. DIC in sepsis is the result of proinflammatory cytokines. There is upregulation of Tissue Factor as well as impairment of anticoagulants and fibrinolysis [1]. Tissue factor activates coagulation, resulting in the deposition of fibrin and hence thrombosis in the microvasculature [1]. The physiologic anticoagulants are consumed by inhibiting the activated coagulation factors [1]. At the same time, the consumption of coagulation factor proteins and platelets leads to occult or clinical bleeding [1].

Another important factor in the pathophysiology of DIC is the consumption of platelets. In the setting of hemothorax or hematoma for example, where there is extensive clot in the body, it is possible to have consumption of platelets and a mild thrombocytopenia. There can be consumption of platelets in retroperitoneal or GI hemorrhage, and bleeding from trauma or surgery [3]. Mild thrombocytopenia can occur with a severe pulmonary embolism [3].

The treatment of DIC is to treat the underlying disorder. If there is no bleeding, then one may simply be observed [1]. If there is clinical bleeding, then the patient may be supported with blood products to correct the lab abnormalities, coagulation tests, hemoglobin and platelets [1]. It is prudent to first confer with one's local blood bank to identify appropriate lab range targets for blood product treatment in the setting of bleeding and no bleeding. If there is active bleeding, a platelet count over 50,000/mm^3 is recommended, as well as an INR and aPTT level less than 1.5 times the control. The INR and aPTT may be corrected with fresh frozen plasma. The INR may be improved with Vitamin K. Fibrinogen should be maintained with cryoprecipitate over 1.5 g/L. If there is traumatic bleeding, it is recommended to keep fibrinogen 1.5 to 2 g per Liter (1). If a patient is stable and does not have DIC, one only needs to keep the platelet count over 10,000/mm^3 [1]. If there is fever, then the platelet count should be over 15,000/mm^3.

Antifibrinolytic agents are contraindicated in DIC, because the fibrinolytic pathway is required to dissolve the widespread fibrin deposition [1]. Heparin treatment remains controversial. There is no evidence to support heparin use in DIC [1]. However, one may be tempted to treat with heparin if the patient manifests more of a thrombotic clinical picture, including limb gangrene.

Dilutional Thrombocytopenia

The diagnosis of dilutional thrombocytopenia occurs when massive blood loss is replaced with red cells that do not have platelets [21]. The clinical presentation needed in order to have dilutional thrombocytopenia is that a patient should have received around 20 units of red cells over 24 hours. The reduction of platelet count is around 50% [2]. The platelet count usually is not less than 50,000/mm^3 [21].

The pathophysiology here is as follows. The replacement of one blood volume within 24 hours may occur after major surgery or trauma, during which time there is consumption of platelets [2]. The treatment is platelet transfusion, which should be given only in those with abnormal bleeding [21].

Mechanical Intravascular Devices - Cardiac Bypass Pump, Intraaortic Balloon Pump

Cardiac Bypass Pump (CBP)

The clinical presentation of thrombocytopenia after heart surgery using cardiac bypass pump is that one can see a 40-60% drop in platelet count on postoperative day 2 or 3 with a subsequent thrombocytosis by day 14 [17]. If platelet count recovery does not occur by day 4, then the thrombocytopenia is likely not due to the pump [14]. The peripheral smear findings in this syndrome may include the presence of some schistocytes.

The pathophysiology of this disorder is that during cardiac surgery, there is thrombocytopenia due to both hemodilution and platelet consumption [17]. The bypass pump is extracorporeal circulation [2]. Usually platelets degranulate and stick to the pump. The cold temperature also destroys the platelets.

The treatment of thrombocytopenia post-CPB is platelet transfusions, which should be reserved for those who are bleeding [21]. If a post-cardiac bypass patient is bleeding but not due to a surgical cause, then a platelet transfusion may help treat the quantitative and qualitative platelet defects [2].

Intraaortic Balloon Pump (IABP)

The intraaortic balloon pump is known to cause thrombocytopenia. Once the device is removed, the thrombocytopenia improves.

Part 2: Thrombocytopenia Present Prior to the Hospitalization

Pseudothrombocytopenia
Thrombotic microangiopathies (TMA): TTP/typical HUS/atypical HUS
Antiphospholipid syndrome (APS)
Evans syndrome
Immune thrombocytopenia – see part 3
Type 2B von Willebrand disease
Congenital thrombocytopenia
Liver disease: hepatitis, hypersplenism, massive splenomegaly
Bone marrow disorders: Myelodysplastic Syndrome, Leukemia, Lymphoma, Multiple Myeloma
Infections obtained prior to hospitalization

Tickborne illness
Bacterial (see Part 1)
Viral (see Part 1)
Recent vaccines
Ingestions: quinine, Schezwan Purpura, alcohol
Vitamin B12 or folate deficiency
Advanced malignancy

Pseudothrombocytopenia

The epidemiology of pseudothrombocytopenia is that once a patient has platelet clumping, they will always have platelet clumping. The diagnosis is made by review of the peripheral smear which will show platelet clumping. As an additional test, one may collect blood in a citrate tube and then check the platelet count. Platelet clumping is a laboratory phenomenon and is of no clinical consequence. The clinical presentation is one in which the patient is usually asymptomatic.

The pathophysiology of this disorder is that there are EDTA dependent platelet antibodies which result in platelet clumping in the test tube. Clumping may occur in any anticoagulant [4}. A blood smear made directly from a finger stick sample would reflect a true platelet count [4]. In this condition, no treatment is indicated.

Thrombotic Microangiopathies (TMA): Thrombocytopenic Thrombotic Purpura (TTP)/Typical Hemolytic Uremic Syndrome (HUS)/Atypical Hemolytic Uremic Syndrome (aHUS)

Thrombotic microangiopathy results in thrombocytopenia, intravascular hemolysis, fragmented red cells, and ischemic organ damage [22, 23]. The peripheral smear findings in TMA include schistocytes (fragmented red cells), a low platelet count, and anisocytosis of red cells. A microangiopathic picture is present where schistocytes are prominent and helmet cells, triangular cells, spherocytes as well as burr cells can be seen [4].

TTP

Most cases of TTP are acquired, whereas the congenital form is due to a mutation in the ADAMTS13 gene, also known as Upshaw-Schulman syndrome [24]. In hereditary TTP the deficiency is due to genetic mutations of ADAMTS13 [22]. Acquired TTP is the result of IgG autoantibodies causing a deficiency in ADAMST13 [22, 25].

The clinical presentation of TTP in adults is as a microangiopathic hemolytic anemia and thrombocytopenia. There should be no other cause of thrombotic microangiopathy and there may also be neurologic abnormalities as well as the possibility of renal failure [24]. The classic pentad includes thrombocytopenia, microangiopathic hemolytic anemia, neurologic and renal abnormalities, and fever [24]. Neurologic abnormalities seen with severe ADAMTS13 deficiency include coma, stroke, seizures, confusion, headache, focal neurologic abnormalities or no neurologic abnormalities [24]. New neurologic abnormalities may occur with treatment [24]. The fever is generally > 37.5 °C. Renal dysfunction can include hematuria and proteinuria as well as acute kidney injury. Gastrointestinal symptoms on presentation include symptoms due to intestinal ischemia like abdominal pain [24].

Many patients have weakness and fatigue, likely due to anemia. Patients also can have bleeding such as easy bruising, petechiae, epistaxis, hematuria, menorrhagia or GI hemorrhage for example [24]. Dyspnea, chest pain, fever and cough are less common [24]. Prior to plasma exchange rarely patients could have acute myocardial infarction, the result of platelet thrombi in the coronary arteries, resulting in sudden death [24].

The pathophysiology here usually involves an unknown trigger that brings about acute disease [22]. Some patients with hereditary deficiency of ADAMTS13 go into clinical remission even with the severe deficiency, thus suggesting a second hit to cause illness [26]. An unknown trigger is also postulated for aHUS [27].

TTP results from a severe deficiency in the von Willebrand factor-cleaving protease, ADAMTS13 (a disintegrin and metalloproteinase with thrombospondin type 1 motif, member 13) [22]. This deficiency is usually caused by an autoantibody to the ADAMTS13 protease [23, 25]. The endothelium releases ultra large von Willebrand factor multimers, which are no longer cleaved by the ADAMTS13 protease [23, 28]. The accumulation of the ultra large multimers in the microcirculation causes shear stress dependent damage to the red cells and platelet aggregation [23]. There is fragmentation of red cells during flow through the high shear, small vessels thus causing a microangiopathic, hemolytic anemia [28]. Consumption of platelets in platelet thrombi results in thrombocytopenia [28]. This can affect the microvasculature of the brain, heart and kidneys [28].

The treatment of choice for TTP is plasma exchange. Plasma exchange removes the autoantibody and repletes ADAMTS13 [28]. Plasma infusion can be given if there is a delay in arranging for plasma exchange [28]. Survival with plasma exchange is 78% [24]. Survival has not changed over the past 20 years [24]. Daily exchange is continued for two days after achieving a normal platelet count, greater than 150,000/mm^3 [28]. The tapering of plasma exchange has not been shown to reduce relapse rates [28].

Patients with progressive neurologic or cardiac symptoms may be increased to twice daily plasma exchange [29]. As an adjunct treatment, corticosteroids such as prednisone or methylprednisolone are given for severe ADAMTS13 deficiency [24]. Corticosteroids are not useful in drug associated TTP or *E. coli* infection [24].

Platelet transfusion is not indicated in TTP simply for a low platelet count [24]. In TTP, platelet transfusion is contraindicated except for life threatening hemorrhage, as the platelet transfusion may cause further thrombotic events [28]. Of note, one published review did not show a detriment to platelet transfusion [24].

Usually one monitors response to plasma exchange by following the platelet count and LDH. The platelet count usually normalizes in a week and responds after the third plasma exchange treatment [24]. The LDH levels are shown to decrease [24]. The anemia takes longer to improve, with renal failure being the sequelae last to recover, with some patients left with renal insufficiency [24]. Once the platelet count is over 50,000/mm^3, it is prudent to start low molecular weight heparin and low dose aspirin [28]. Packed red blood cell transfusion and folic acid are given to support the patient during hemolysis [28]. Usually one keeps the hemoglobin greater than 7 g/dL but a higher level may be prudent if there is evidence of cardiac problems [28]. Once the platelet counts are normal for two days, then plasma exchange is stopped, but the prednisone is usually continued [24]. An exacerbation of TTP can occur two weeks after stopping plasma exchange [24]. A frequent complication of plasma exchange is catheter-related sepsis [24], which in itself can exacerbate TTP.

There was a phase II study that supported adding rituximab within 3 days of admission for acute TTP to standard therapy with plasma exchange and steroids for patients with idiopathic TTP [29]. Patients were then given weekly rituximab for 4 to 8 times and this showed a reduction in relapse rate [29]. One should wait 4 hours after rituximab to start plasma exchange [28]. Traditionally, rituximab has been used to treat patients who develop an exacerbation after a response or a relapse after remission [24]. Plasma exchange can be done twice daily if the patient is refractory and or critically ill. In this small group of patients with TTP, once they improve, the frequency of plasma exchange can then be decreased to once a day [24].

Rituximab is an anti CD-20 antibody that depletes B cells [29]. It is used as a second line treatment in patients that do not respond to plasma exchange or steroids [29]. Rituximab has also been used in cases of relapsed idiopathic TTP patients with a previously demonstrated antibody to ADAMTS13 who electively choose to take rituximab to prevent further relapses [29]. In refractory and relapsing TTP, further immunosuppressive treatments including cyclophosphamide, vincristine, and cyclosporine have also been used [24, 29].

For congenital TTP, treatment includes plasma infusion/exchange or use of virally-inactivated intermediate purity factor VIII concentrate containing ADAMTS13 [28]. Some patients require regular therapy to maintain platelet count and avoid relapses, whereas other mildly affected patients only require occasional treatment [28]. For congenital TTP, molecular diagnostic testing of siblings and first-degree relatives is recommended [28]. Patients can have a homozygous or compound heterozygote defect in ADAMST13 [28].

The prognosis of TTP prior to plasma exchange was very poor with mortality rates of about 90%. However, with plasma exchange, the mortality has decreased to 20% [30]. The risk for relapse is most common during the first year of recovery [24]. TTP as we know it consists of acute episodes of microvascular thrombosis [30]. Therefore, recovery from an acute episode may be complete, but patients remain at risk for recurrent episodes [30]. Some long term consequences that TTP patients have reported include inability to concentrate, forgetfulness, and overall less endurance [24].

In one described TTP cohort, there was increased morbidity and mortality noted. The lifetime prevalence of SLE was higher than in the general population, at 14% [30]. Hypertension and depression were also more common in survivors of TTP [30]. Another observation was the presence of a greater BMI in their cohort [30]. ADAMTS13 deficiency during remission may be a risk factor for both cardiovascular and cerebrovascular disease [30]. It is postulated that the diagnosis of TTP may be an opportunity for primary care physicians to combat the public health problems of obesity, hypertension, depression, and SLE [30]. Of note, glomerular filtration rate (GFR) was not different between TTP survivors and normal controls [30].

Typical HUS

HUS may be defined as microangiopathic hemolytic anemia, thrombocytopenia, and renal failure [27]. This syndrome follows enterohemorrhagic *Escherichia coli* infection, usually occurring in children [22]. It is a TMA with renal impairment, occurring with Shiga toxin producing organisms such as *Escherichia coli* and *Shigella dysenteriae* [25].

The epidemiology of TMA is such that risk factors include genetic disorders, autoimmune disease, and cancer [22]. The thrombotic microangiopathies have also been associated with hematopoietic stem cell transplant, pregnancy, HIV, infection, and drugs such as mitomycin C, quinine, and ticlopidine [26]. The incidence of TTP is 4 to 6 cases per million of the population per year in the United States [28].

Ninety percent of the shiga toxin associated HUS occurs in children [23]. Ten percent of HUS is atypical HUS, caused by complement dysregulation [27]. Half of patients with aHUS do not have an identifiable complement mutation [25].

It is important not to miss the diagnosis of TTP, as TTP is a medical emergency and if left untreated, the mortality is 90% without plasma exchange [28]. The initial diagnosis is based on history, physical exam, lab values, and peripheral smear review [28].

It is important to order ADAMTS13 activity with reflex inhibitor in the blood before the first plasma exchange [24]. Severe deficiency is defined as less than 10% normal [24]. One does not wait for the level prior to starting plasma exchange and even patients with mild deficiency may benefit from plasma exchange [24].

In acquired TTP, ADAMTS13 activity is less than 10% and there is an antibody inhibitor [25]. In congenital TTP, usually ADAMTS 13 activity is less than 5% and there are no antibodies [25]. Molecular diagnosis to find a defect in ADAMTS13 may be performed [28].

Laboratory results show anemia, elevated LDH, and acute renal failure [24]. Usually the platelet count is $10{,}000/mm^3$-$30{,}000/mm^3$ [28]. Hemoglobin usually is 8 g/dl-10 g/dl. Labs show low haptoglobin, an elevated reticulocyte count, an elevated LDH, and a negative direct Coombs test [28]. The INR, aPTT and fibrinogen are normal [28]. The D-dimer as well is usually normal. The troponin I may be elevated. Heart failure is more common in those who have received a platelet transfusion [28]. On presentation, it is important to test for HIV, hepatitis B and C infections, and to perform a pregnancy test.

The clinical presentation of typical HUS is usually in children who present with abdominal pain, bloody diarrhea, microangiopathic hemolytic anemia, thrombocytopenia, and renal failure [22, 24]. It is associated with *E. coli* 0157:H7 Shiga toxin producing infection (24). The clinical course is usually one episode [24]. In typical HUS, renal failure is more predominant and there are less neurologic symptoms [23, 28]. There was a reported *E. coli* outbreak where neurologic symptoms were delayed and developed after the second week of illness once diarrhea resolved. The neurological symptoms were felt to be autoimmune in etiology [23].

The pathophysiology of typical HUS is that the Shiga toxin stimulates the release of ultra large von Willebrand factor multimers from endothelial cells and the result is the activation of platelets [23]. Shiga toxin inhibits ADAMTS13 function, resulting in accumulation of large vWF multimers [23]. Von Willebrand factor concentrations are altered.

The treatment for typical HUS in adults is plasma exchange, because at the time of initial treatment the cause is usually not clear [24]. Missing the diagnosis of TTP can result in permanent neurologic and renal sequelae along with a high mortality [24]. Diarrhea associated HUS is usually treated with supportive care and at times can require hemodialysis [28].

The prognosis for typical HUS is favorable with only about 25% of patients left with any type of renal dysfunction [27]. Shiga toxin associated HUS also has a favorable outcome.

Atypical HUS

It is very important to distinguish atypical HUS from TTP [25]. There is no diagnostic test to confirm the diagnosis [25]. The diagnosis may be made by finding a mutation of one or more of the complement proteins including complement factor H (CFH), CFI, C3, CFB, thrombomodulin, membrane cofactor protein (MCP), but only half of patients carry these mutations [25]. A CFH autoantibody test could also be ordered [25]. Another way to diagnose atypical HUS is by monitoring the initial response to plasma exchange over the first five days [25]. If the pre-treatment ADAMTS13 activity is not severely low, then one could consider aHUS. If there is only partial hematologic remission and renal worsening, then one may consider aHUS.

If ADAMTS13 is less than 10% and there is response to plasma exchange, then the diagnosis is TTP [25]. If ADAMTS13 is deficient and renal function worsens, then one must use intensive immunosuppressive therapy [25]. If there is a response to plasma exchange and ADAMTS13 is greater than 10%, then the diagnosis is aHUS responsive to plasma exchange [25]. Then one would obtain complement mutation studies [25]. If the ADAMTS13 is not deficient and renal function worsens, then consider aHUS. Then one would stop treatment with plasma exchange and start eculizumab [25].

The differential diagnosis of TMA includes other disorders that cause thrombotic microangiopathy include infection, malignancy, and malignant hypertension. Other causes of TMAs include glomerulopathies and viral infections, including HIV and influenza [25].

Autoimmune disorders such as Systemic Lupus Erythematosus (SLE) and the antiphospholipid antibody syndrome may also cause TMA [24]. If another reason for the TMA is found, then plasma exchange is stopped [24].

The clinical course of atypical HUS is that of recurrent HUS episodes [24]. Atypical HUS usually has no diarrhea. It is very important to distinguish atypical HUS from TTP, and many symptoms overlap. GI symptoms can be seen in aHUS and TTP [25]. Neurologic injury can be seen in both aHUS and TTP [25]. Renal injury in TTP requiring hemodialysis occurs in less than 10% of patients, whereas in aHUS, acute renal failure requiring hemodialysis is a prominent clinical feature [25]. Atypical HUS also has microangiopathic hemolytic anemia, thrombocytopenia, and acute renal failure [27].

The pathophysiology in atypical HUS is the result of complement dysregulation and overactivation due to complement gene mutations or CFH autoantibodies [22, 24, 25]. Fifty percent of the mutations are in genes that regulate complement. As a result of activation of complement, there is microvascular injury and activation of platelets, coagulation, and leukocytes [25].

Thrombomodulin is located in the vasculature, and plays a role in coagulation, immunity, and complement activation [27]. Thrombomodulin negatively regulates complement by accelerating inactivation of C3b [27]. Variants in the gene encoding thrombomodulin predisposes to endothelial injury and microvascular thrombosis [27]. Five percent of cases of mutations in thrombomodulin are associated with atypical HUS [27]. In addition to the mutation in the allele, viral illness, environmental, genetic and epigenetic factors may be requisite for causing disease [27].

The treatment for suspected TTP/aHUS initially is plasma exchange [25]. Plasma exchange induces a remission in varying rates from 25 to 88% [25]. It is important to obtain pretreatment ADAMTS13 activity and CFH autoantibodies when the diagnosis of aHUS is entertained [25]. Assessment of response to plasma exchange over the first 5 days is critical

[25]. Stabilization of the serum creatinine should be seen over the first 5 days, and if ADAMST13 activity is less than 10%, one should think of TTP [25]. ADAMTS13 over 10% and improvement with treatment makes the diagnosis of aHUS [25]. ADAMTS13 over 10% but unable to stop plasma exchange also supports the diagnosis of aHUS [25]. Patients with a hematologic response and worsening renal injury could also have aHUS but a case that is not responding to plasma exchange. In cases not responding to plasma exchange, then eculizumab should be started [25].

Eculizumab is the treatment for atypical HUS [28]. It is an inhibitor of terminal complement activation [25]. It binds to C5 and prevents activation of C5 that leads to the formation of the membrane attack complex [25]. The sooner eculizumab is started, the better the improvement in renal function [25]. Two weeks prior to treatment with eculizumab, the meningococcal vaccine should be administered [25]. If one cannot wait two weeks to start the drug, then prophylactic antibiotic therapy for meningococcus is given in conjunction with the vaccine [25]. In patients responding to plasma exchange, then the plasma therapy should be tapered and the treatment individualized. For patients whose aHUS is caused by a CFH autoantibody, the treatment is long term plasma exchange and immunosuppressive therapy [25]. Immunosuppressive therapy includes steroids, azathioprine, mycophenolate mofetil, cyclophosphamide, and rituximab [25].

An anti-CFH antibody titer may help guide therapy [25]. If the patient does not respond to eculizumab after 8 weeks, then the diagnosis of aHUS must be reconsidered [25].

The prognosis for atypical HUS, whether familial or sporadic, is poor as it is an aggressive disease. It usually recurs, with a rate of 50% for end stage renal failure and a 25% mortality rate [27]. If the patient is found to have a membrane cofactor protein (MCP) mutation, the prognosis however is good.

Special Categories of TTP

Hematopoietic Stem Cell Transplantation-Associated TMA

There is no ADAMTS13 deficiency in this disorder characterized by rare neurologic symptoms and a lack of systemic microthrombi formation. It is postulated to be due to endothelial toxicity due to chemotherapy, infections, immunosuppressive medication and graft-versus-host disease [28]. Plasma exchange is not an effective treatment in this disease [24].

Drug Associated TTP

Less than 15% of all TTP cases are due to drugs [28]. The drug is taken before the diagnosis, and there is an acute immune mediated reaction that occurs that causes the clinical syndrome [24].

Quinine associated TTP presents with sudden onset of chills, fever, nausea, vomiting, diarrhea, and acute renal failure several hours after ingestion of quinine or tonic water [24]. TTP associated with chemotherapy and calcineurin inhibitors presents with gradual renal failure and TMA [24].

TTP may be associated with clopidogrel as well as ticlopidine. Simvastatin, trimethoprim and pegylated interferon have been reported in antibody positive TTP [28].

Drugs Associated with HUS

The most common associated with HUS are gemcitabine, bleomycin, and mitomycin-C.

HIV Associated TTP

TTP may be the presenting feature of HIV or can be seen in those patients with low CD4 counts who are also non-compliant with antiretroviral therapy [28].

The treatment here is with Highly Active Antiretroviral Therapy (HAART) and plasma exchange (Scully and 1). HAART therapy helps improve the immune system of the patient and prevent TTP relapse [28].

Malignancy Associated TMA

This disorder can present in an early stage of cancer or in the case of disseminated disease. ADAMTS13 activity is not significantly reduced [28]. Plasma exchange is not helpful and treatment of the cancer is recommended [28].

Pancreatitis Associated TTP

This disease has been well described in the literature. It can occur several days after recovery from pancreatitis. ADAMTS13 activity generally does not correlate with the severity of the TTP or the pancreatitis. All patients with pancreatitis associated TTP were treated with plasma exchange and steroids [28].

Antiphospholipid Syndrome (APS)

The epidemiology of APS is such that the thrombocytopenia prevalence in the antiphospholipid syndrome is between 30 to 46 percent [31].

The diagnosis and clinical presentation should be discussed. The APS is an autoimmune disease associated with arterial and venous thrombosis, recurrent fetal loss and antiphospholipid antibodies [32]. The Sapporo Antiphospholipid Syndrome criteria include thrombosis and pregnancy morbidity [31]. Two or more positive antibody determinations are required 12 weeks apart, anticardiolipin IgG or IgM, β_2 glycoprotein I Ab IgG or IgM, and the lupus anticoagulant [31].

The APS may be associated with thrombocytopenia or autoimmune hemolytic anemia [31]. However, antiphospholipid antibodies and cytopenias without thrombosis or pregnancy morbidity cannot be classified as the APS syndrome [31]. The hematologic manifestations may predate the clinical manifestations and one study reported that 60% of antiphospholipid antibody positive patients with ITP developed thrombosis in 5 years of follow up [31].

There is the thought that cytopenias, including thrombocytopenia or autoimmune hemolytic anemia, constitute a distinct subset of patients with the antiphospholipid syndrome [31]. Hematologic Antiphospholipid Syndrome (APS) refers to the patient who continues to have cytopenia as clinical manifestations without the development of thrombosis and in the absence of the clinical and serologic features of SLE [31]. Half of antiphospholipid antibody positive patients with thrombocytopenia eventually develop antiphospholipid syndrome and half of these patients remain free of symptoms of APS [31].

Primary antiphospholipid syndrome can evolve into systemic lupus erythematosus (SLE) [31]. SLE patients with low platelets have been found to have greater levels of IgG anticardiolipin antibody [31]. Triple positivity, the combination of positive anticardiolipin antibodies, lupus anticoagulant, and anti-β_2 glycoprotein I antibodies is strongly associated with adverse clinical outcomes [33].

The pathophysiology of APS is that the antiphospholipid antibodies are a family of antibodies that react with serum phospholipid binding plasma proteins [32]. The autoantibody binds to the activated platelets via β_2-glycoprotein I [31]. Patients with anti-β_2 glycoprotein I antibodies are at high risk for thrombosis [31]. The treatment here is that if thrombosis is present, lifelong anticoagulation therapy is recommended.

Evans Syndrome

The epidemiology of Evans syndrome is that it has a prevalence of 10% as a manifestation of the primary antiphospholipid syndrome [31]. The diagnosis is considered when a patient has an autoimmune hemolytic anemia (AIHA) and ITP simultaneously or being sequentially diagnosed with both diseases [34]. To diagnose the hemolytic anemia, one must demonstrate an elevated reticulocyte count, increased indirect bilirubin and elevated LDH, a low haptoglobin, and a positive Coombs test [34].

The clinical presentation can be quite variable and depends upon the level of anemia and thrombocytopenia. The peripheral smear findings in Evans syndrome are spherocytes and a low platelet count.

The pathophysiology of Evans syndrome is presence of both ITP and autoimmune hemolytic anemia. There is antibody mediated destruction of the red cells and platelets [34]. The treatment in this disorder is the use of corticosteroids as first line [34]. Splenectomy is another option to consider and rituximab has been used successfully. Usually the response to rituximab in Evans Syndrome is seen in either ITP or AIHA, but not both [34].

Immune Thrombocytopenia: See Part 3

Type 2B Von Willebrand Disease

The epidemiology of Type 2B von Willebrand Disease is that it is inherited in autosomal dominant pattern. In order to make the diagnosis, it is important to ask the patient about a personal history of bleeding and a family history of bleeding. Pertinent questions include abnormal bleeding with prior procedures, dental work, surgeries, heavy menses, and spontaneous bruising. It is important to ask about the timing of bleeding, the necessity of blood transfusion after surgery, dental extraction, trauma, menses, and childbirth [35]. It is also important to elicit medication and herbal medication history.

To make the diagnosis, one must first obtain a CBC, INR, aPTT, and a fibrinogen level. The aPTT is often normal in Type 2B von Willebrand Disease [35]. Laboratory tests to order include Factor VIII assay, von Willebrand Factor antigen and a VWF ristocetin cofactor activity which shows the plasma's ability to agglutinate platelets in the presence of ristocetin [35]. A low-dose ristocetin-induced platelet aggregation test (LD-RIPA) identifies increased binding between VWF and platelets [35]. The collagen-binding assay measures the binding of large VWF multimers to collagen, and is another way to measure the functional activity of the molecule [35]. One should also order VWF multimers [35].

In Type 2B von Willebrand disease, there is a low VWF ristocetin cofactor activity, enhanced LD-RIPA, and mild thrombocytopenia [35]. The LD-RIPA test is used to enhance platelet agglutination in the presence of gain-of function mutations [35].

The clinical presentation of Type 2B von Willebrand Disease requires a good history as patients may have a personal or family history of easy bruising and bleeding [1]. It is possible at times to have a late presentation of an inherited bleeding disorder. Usually the patient presents with persistent oozing after an injury or surgery [1]. The findings in the peripheral smear are normal with a platelet count that may be normal or low.

The pathophysiology of Type 2B von Willebrand Disease involves understanding a little about Von Willebrand factor (VWF) itself. VWF is a large, multimeric glycoprotein that promotes platelet adhesion to the exposed subendothelium [35]. It helps with platelet aggregation and chaperones factor VIII in the plasma and protects it from proteolytic degradation [35]. VWF is synthesized in the vascular endothelium [35].

Type 2B von Willebrand Disease is a qualitative defect in VWF. The qualitative defect is due to gain of function mutation in VWF at the binding site for GP1bA, which results in rapid clearance of the platelet/VWF complex [35]. Type 2B is a gain of function mutation resulting in spontaneous VWF-platelet binding under physiologic shear conditions, leading to clearance of the highest molecular weight multimers and a mild thrombocytopenia [35].

The treatment of this disorder, since the molecular defect is in the VWF molecule, is with VWF concentrates, such as Humate-P [35].

Congenital Thrombocytopenia

The epidemiology of congenital thrombocytopenia is such that it is a very rare condition [21]. Patients are often misdiagnosed as having ITP [2]. One needs to consider the diagnosis of congenital thrombocytopenia in a patient with a family history of thrombocytopenia, or a patient with presumed ITP that does not respond to therapy [2]. Anatomic abnormalities and abnormal peripheral smear may support the diagnosis [2]. Genetic diagnosis should be obtained if feasible [2].

Clinically, congenital thrombocytopenia can be diagnosed in infancy or even in adulthood [4]. Older patients are often misdiagnosed as ITP and are treated inappropriately [4]. Family studies may be helpful in obtaining the diagnosis [4]. The diagnosis should be suspected in children with chronic refractory ITP [4]. The peripheral smear findings in this disorder are the presence of giant platelets [4].

The pathophysiology of congenital thrombocytopenia is multifactorial and pathogenesis is dependent upon the patient's underlying condition. The treatment is platelet transfusion if required for bleeding or surgical procedures [21].

Unnecessary platelet transfusion could lead to alloimmunization, and then when a platelet transfusion is needed, the platelet count may not increase appropriately [21].

Liver Disease: Hepatitis, Hypersplenism

The epidemiology of thrombocytopenia in liver disease is that thrombocytopenia may be seen in chronic liver disease and is actually relatively common [36]. Seventy six percent of patients with cirrhosis have thrombocytopenia [36]. The degree of thrombocytopenia correlates with the severity of liver disease [36].

The diagnosis is made rather easily because the liver synthesizes thrombopoietin and coagulation factors (except factor VIII). Reduced synthetic function of the liver may cause an elevation of INR more than aPTT, in addition to thrombocytopenia [1].

The clinical presentation is worth discussing. The reduction in coagulation factors and anticoagulants is balanced, such that thrombosis does not occur and thrombin generation is normal [1]. Usually a platelet count from hypersplenism is not below 50,000/mm^3.

The peripheral smear findings could be variable. White cells might be decreased and the platelets are usually decreased. Red cell morphology may show macrocytes, target cells, acanthocytes, and polychromatophilia [37].

The pathophysiology of thrombocytopenia seen in liver disease involves many mechanisms for the thrombocytopenia, including portal hypertension [38]. Hypersplenism may cause sequestration of platelets in the spleen. Other possibilities include decreased thrombopoietin production and viruses that could cause bone marrow suppression [38].

The treatment principle here is that in general, one does not need to treat the thrombocytopenia or a prolonged INR/aPTT if there is no bleeding [1]. Vitamin K may be given to help aid in the synthesis of coagulation factors with variable success [1].

The treatment of thrombocytopenia prior to initiation of viral hepatitis C therapy is worth discussing. Eltrombopag is a small molecule, nonpeptide oral platelet growth factor and works as a thrombopoietin receptor agonist [38]. It causes proliferation and differentiation of megakaryocytes, thereby increasing platelet production [38]. Patients are usually eligible for antiviral therapy when platelets are greater than 70,000/mm^3 or 100,000/mm^3, depending on the type of antiviral treatment. Many patients with hepatitis C have a lower platelet count. Eltrombopag was used for the first 12 weeks of antiviral treatment and was shown to increase the platelet count in hepatitis C cirrhosis patients, thereby allowing initiation of antiviral therapy [38]. The most common side effects of this treatment included headache, dry mouth, abdominal pain, and nausea [38]. Careful consideration should be given prior to administering this medication to patients at risk for VTE or in those where the hepatic toxicity could put the patient at risk for further harm.

The treatment of patients with liver disease prior to procedures is a common clinical question posed to the physician. At times, patients with liver disease require procedures and it would be of benefit to have the platelet count a bit higher. There was a study to test eltrombopag before procedures in patients with cirrhosis and thrombocytopenia [36]. It was found that even though eltrombopag reduced the need for platelet transfusions, it was associated with an increased risk of portal vein thrombosis [36]. As such, eltrombopag is not recommended as an alternative to platelet transfusion in patients with chronic liver disease and thrombocytopenia undergoing elective invasive procedures [36].

In a patient with cirrhosis and thrombocytopenia, one may consider a platelet transfusion prior to a procedure to reduce the risk of bleeding [36]. If the platelet count is less than 50,000/mm^3 a platelet transfusion may be administered. For platelet counts between 50,000/mm^3 to 80,000/mm^3, the decision to administer platelet transfusion is subjective [36] and may ultimately dependent upon the type of procedure to be performed.

Massive Splenomegaly

The diagnosis of thrombocytopenia in the setting of massive splenomegaly is seen with the appropriate physical examination or radiographic findings and usually the platelet count is not below 30,000/mm^3 [21].

The underlying pathophysiology in massive splenomegaly is that there is sequestration of platelets in the spleen which communicate with the platelets in the circulation [21]. Patients with hepatic cirrhosis also have a deficiency in thrombopoietin, which also contributes to the cause of the thrombocytopenia [21].

The treatment for thrombocytopenia associated with massive splenomegaly involves consideration that for procedures and surgery sometimes a higher platelet count is needed. It could take considerable amount of platelets at times to increase the platelet count to the desired level. Platelet transfusion may be given prior to procedures or surgery realizing that there will not be a significant increase in the platelet count. Rarely a splenectomy is considered [21].

Bone Marrow Disorders: Myelodysplastic Syndrome (MDS), Leukemia, Lymphoma, Multiple Myeloma

The epidemiology of thrombocytopenia varies with the disorder. Thrombocytopenia may the presenting sign of a bone marrow disorder. Usually patients would have some constitutional symptoms like fever, night sweats, and weight loss. The physical examination may show lymphadenopathy or splenomegaly. In these disorders, usually the other bone marrow cell lines in the CBC are affected, not just the platelet count.

In MDS one would often have anemia with a low platelet count [39]. Low grade lymphoid neoplasms and lymphoproliferative disorders may also present with thrombocytopenia [40].

The pathophysiology of the thrombocytopenia seen in bone marrow disorders is disease dependent. For example, in AML and MDS, there is ineffective hematopoiesis and a hematopoiesis suppressing bone marrow microenvironment by the malignant clone [39]. Acute leukemia patients may also have DIC as an explanation for the thrombocytopenia. For example, in acute myelogenous leukemia (AML), some 14-30% of the patients have bleeding due to thrombocytopenia [39]. In chronic lymphocytic leukemia, thrombocytopenia may be from bone marrow infiltration or autoimmune phenomenon.

The peripheral smear finding in bone marrow disorders can be rouleaux formation in multiple myeloma, an example of a dysproteinemia [4]. With the presence of a leukemia and MDS, one may see abnormal leukocytes [4].

Infections Obtained Prior to Hospitalization

Tickborne Illness

The epidemiology of the various tickborne illnesses varies, for example, Babesiosis occurs more frequently in the immunocompromised and those over age 50. The diagnosis of these types of infections can be made in some instances by sending serologies, as is the case with Lyme disease, Rocky Mountain spotted fever, ehrlichiosis, and anaplasmosis [41]. The reverse-transcription polymerase chain reaction for human granulocytic anaplasmosis (HGA) is another test to consider ordering [41]. Anaplasmosis antibodies take 2 – 3 weeks to become positive and may not be helpful in the acute setting [41].

The clinical presentation is commonly that there would be no prior history of thrombocytopenia in the patient. In HGA, there is thrombocytopenia, transaminitis, and history of a tick bite. With effective antibiotic treatment, there is resolution of the thrombocytopenia, fever, transaminitis, and confusion [41].

Babesia microti can present with hemolytic anemia and thrombocytopenia [26]. Patients may have mental status change, weakness, disorientation, and diarrhea [26]. The clinical course can last as long as two weeks [26].

The peripheral smear finding in human granulocytic anaplasmosis (HGA) is the presence of morulae inside neutrophils. One must carefully look for inclusion bodies in white blood cells and in monocytes [41]. Please see a photo demonstrating this finding from the ASH Image Bank (http://imagebank.hematology.org, ASH Image Bank; 2013-0023065).

In Babesiosis, there may be parasites both inside and outside of the red cells. [26] Please see an example of this finding as seen from the ASH Image Bank (http://imagebank.hematology.org, ASH Image Bank; 2014-26965). There could also be mild neutropenia and evidence of hemolytic anemia on the peripheral smear [37].

The pathophysiology in rickettsial infections is that platelets may be consumed in vasculitic lesions [2]. The treatment of Anaplasmosis is with intravenous doxycycline. Babesiosis is treated with a combination of two types of anti-parasitic medications, atovaquone plus a macrolide agent.

Recent Vaccines

A transient thrombocytopenia can develop in children or adults after vaccination [8]. There has been an association of measles-mumps-rubella vaccine and ITP in children [42]. The MMR vaccine was associated with ITP in 0.87 to 4 cases per 100,000 vaccine doses [43]. The incidence of ITP after measles or rubella infection is even higher at 6 to 1200 per 100,000 cases [43]. In Taiwan, there was a case-control study showing a potential association between ITP and influenza vaccine [42]. Based on another case-control study, in general, there was no definite connection between the incidences of ITP with vaccination in adults [42].

Ingestions

Ingestions may also cause a drug induced thrombocytopenia, and the list includes herbal remedies and foods [8].

Quinine Induced Thrombocytopenia (QITP)

The epidemiology of QITP came about because Quinine was used as an antimalarial drug and is now used to treat nocturnal muscle cramps [8]. Quinine is in tonic water, and the resultant immune thrombocytopenia is referred to as cocktail purpura [8]. The clinical presentation of QITP is that it can cause a severe thrombocytopenia of less than 10,000/mm^3 [7]. The physical examination may reveal petechiae or mucosal bleeding. There is usually the abrupt onset of thrombocytopenia after an inconsistent period of time of taking quinine [7].

The pathophysiology of QITP includes peripheral platelet destruction and inhibition of proplatelet and platelet production by megakaryocytes along with the presence of immunoglobulins against VWF or fibrinogen receptors GPIb/IX or GPIIb/IIIa [7]. Since megakaryocytes also express GPIb/IX and GPIIb/IIIa as a late marker, the antibodies interact with megakaryocytes and cause apoptosis [7]. Late megakaryocytes are thus decreased in number [7]. The treatment in QITP is cessation of the drug and or the avoidance of tonic water. It usually takes 5 to 10 days for the platelet count to return to normal [7]. This is the time needed for the megakaryocytes to repopulate the bone marrow [7].

Schezwan Purpura

Schezwan Purpura was described in a laboratory technologist who used his platelets as a control in experiments on platelet aggregation [44]. He usually had normal platelet aggregation. The morning after eating a large quantity of Schezwanese hot bean curd, he was found to have a platelet aggregation abnormality [44]. He had mild bruising and bleeding symptoms. Mo-er or Black Tree Fungus is a common ingredient in Schezwan Chinese food [44]. It was determined that ingestion of mo-er was shown to inhibit platelet function [44]. It may be prudent to counsel patients with low platelet counts or plasma coagulation disorders to avoid mo-er, which could theoretically increase bleeding risk.

Alcohol

Acute alcohol toxicity may cause thrombocytopenia. It also inhibits platelet aggregation [1].

Vitamin B12 or Folate Deficiency

Vitamin B12 deficiency which is seen in pernicious anemia can be associated with thrombocytopenia that resolves with Vitamin B12 replacement. As well, acute folate deficiency may also present with thrombocytopenia. The peripheral smear findings here are consistent with a megaloblastic picture and include neutrophil hypersegmentation, macrocytosis as well as oval macrocytes [4]. Thrombocytopenia may also be present.

Advanced Malignancy

Thrombocytopenia may also present in advanced malignancy. Clinically, it can present as bone marrow infiltration by metastatic cells which can cause anemia or any pancytopenia for that matter. Advanced malignancies may also cause a compensated chronic DIC with slightly elevated INR, aPTT, accompanied by a slightly low fibrinogen, and slightly decreased platelet count. The peripheral smear findings here include a normal to low platelet count, which could also be microangiopathic or myelophthisic. Myelophthisic anemia is "anemia or pancytopenia" associated with marrow infiltration by tumor [4]. There could be the presence of anisocytosis, poikilocytosis, schistocytes, tear drop cells, nucleated red cells, and immature neutrophils on the peripheral smear [4]. The platelet count in this condition may be normal or low. The pathophysiology here is quite simple and the problem is caused by bone marrow infiltration of tumor cells. Another mechanism to explain the thrombocytopenia is the presence of a chronic, low grade DIC. The treatment of choice here is to treat the underlying malignancy.

Part 3: Causes for a Platelet Count Less Than 10,000/mm^3

ITP – immune thrombocytopenia

Drug induced thrombocytopenia: Glycoprotein IIb/IIIa antagonists

Post-transfusion purpura – see part 1
Disseminated intravascular coagulation (DIC) – see part 1

Immune Thrombocytopenia (ITP)

The epidemiology of ITP is discussed in more detail in another chapter in this book. From 1928-1989, the mortality rate of newly diagnosed ITP was 2.1% and from 1973 to 2004 it decreased to 0.8% [43]. The mortality rate of chronic ITP varies from 5.4 – 6.6% [43].

Patients over the age of 60 with a platelet count of less than 30,000/mm^3 have an increased risk of bleeding, with a 5 year fatal bleeding risk of 48%. For patients under age 40, this bleeding risk is much lower, at 2.2% [43]. The definition of ITP is based upon the fact that patients of non-Western ethnicities may have a normal baseline platelet count between 100,000/mm^3-150,000/mm^3 [43]. As such, primary ITP is defined by a platelet count of less than 100,000/mm^3 [43].

ITP definitions:

- Newly diagnosed – up to 3 months from diagnosis [43]
- Persistent – 3 to 12 months from diagnosis [43]
- Chronic – lasting more than 12 months since diagnosis [43]
- Refractory – the presence of severe ITP after splenectomy [43]
- Severe – clinically relevant bleeding to need treatment or the occurrence of new bleeding symptoms to require more intervention [43]

Primary immune thrombocytopenia (ITP) is defined as an isolated thrombocytopenia in the absence of any cause [43]. Secondary immune thrombocytopenia has been associated with various infections, including *Helicobacter pylori*, hepatitis C virus, and HIV [42].

Immune thrombocytopenia has also been associated with autoimmune disease and the antiphospholipid antibody syndrome [43]. Drug induced thrombocytopenia must also be excluded [43]. Common variable immunodeficiency (CVID) patients also have an increased incidence of ITP [45]. For a more extensive discussion about the causes of secondary ITP, please see the chapter entitled "Immune Thrombocytopenic Purpura in Adults" contained in this book.

The diagnosis of ITP may be difficult to make. There is no one particular diagnostic test of choice [43]. A CBC with differential and peripheral smear should always be obtained. If a patient presents with typical ITP, a bone marrow biopsy is not necessary [43]. Any abnormalities in the CBC except for the presence of a microcytic anemia due to iron deficiency should be investigated with a bone marrow biopsy [43]. The bone marrow biopsy in ITP shows normal or increased megakaryocytes, the absence of dysplastic changes on morphology, and no abnormal cytogenetics associated with myelodysplasia [34].

At present, antiphospholipid antibodies and antinuclear antibody testing is not recommended [43]. At diagnosis, it is important to exclude secondary causes and for this reason, HIV and hepatitis C testing is recommended [43]. Hepatitis B testing may also be useful as these patients can develop portal hypertension and cirrhosis, leading to thrombocytopenia as well. An abdominal sonogram may also be helpful in finding a secondary cause of ITP [46].

The clinical presentation is based upon the natural history of ITP, which is that spontaneous remission does occur anywhere from 6 months to 3 years, but is less common in adults [43]. The clinical course is one of relapses and remissions over many years [43]. There have been a few cases of a relapse of ITP in the setting of infections, such as influenza A virus infection [42]. The history and physical examination may show evidence of bleeding [43]. If during the course of treatment for typical ITP other features like an abnormal WBC count, lymphadenopathy or multiple cytopenias develop, then one must reassess the diagnosis of ITP [43].

The peripheral smear findings in ITP show that the platelet count is low. Moderately enlarged platelets are the hallmark finding in this disorder [4]. The peripheral smear may also be normal to variable. There may also be evidence of simultaneous iron deficiency.

The pathophysiology of ITP warrants a brief discussion. There is an immune destruction of normal platelets in response to an unknown stimulus [43, 48]. The accelerated clearance and destruction of antibody-coated platelets by tissue macrophages occurs mainly in the spleen [40]. Due to the accelerated clearance, plasma thrombopoietin level may be normal to minimally elevated [40]. Platelet production is also decreased [43, 45]. Chronic ITP antibodies target antigens on megakaryocytes and proplatelets and inhibit the production and maturation of megakaryocytes [7, 40].

Treatment should be reserved for those patients who are at risk for bleeding [40]. This cut-off level is deemed to be a platelet count of less than 30,000/mm^3 [43]. The decision to treat is based on the severity of bleeding, risk of bleeding which takes into account prior bleeding episodes in a patient, hypertension, older age, comorbidities, side effects of treatment, the activity level of the patient which includes sports, and patient preference [40, 43].

First line treatment for symptomatic ITP is glucocorticoids [46]. Prednisone at 1 mg/kg by mouth daily is a standard first line treatment. Complete remission with oral prednisone occurs in around 10-30% of patients [40]. Another acceptable option is a short course of dexamethasone 40 mg daily for 4 days [43]. This short course may be repeated [43]. Studies of high dose, pulsed dexamethasone have a complete remission rate of 60-80%, but these trials need to be confirmed [40]. At present high dose dexamethasone is not considered superior to prednisone [40]. Longer courses of steroids, such as prednisone 1 mg/kg oral for 21 days and then tapered off has been favored because there is a longer time to loss of response [43]. There was a study in newly diagnosed ITP where the addition of rituximab to high dose dexamethasone showed an improved response of 63% compared to 36% without rituximab. However, it is unclear how this compares to prolonged corticosteroids [43]. Risks with rituximab therapy include fulminant hepatitis B reactivation and progressive multifocal leukoencephalopathy [40].

If one wants to increase the platelet count rapidly, then intravenous immunoglobulin (IVIG) is another option. The initial dose recommended is 1 gram/kg as a one-time dose, and may be repeated to a total of 2 g/kg if no response [43]. Rh positive nonsplenectomized patients may receive WinRho, but there must be careful monitoring for life threatening hemolysis [43]. The use of intravenous immunoglobulin in combination with oral prednisone as first line treatment for severe ITP gives a more sustained and rapid short-term response [46]. One may use IVIG or WinRho alone if corticosteroids are contraindicated [43].

In chronic ITP, patients are often observed because the side effects of treatment may be worse than the risk of bleeding [47]. The goal of treatment is a platelet count that prevents bleeding [43]. The treatment of ITP using splenectomy removes the primary site of platelet destruction and the spleen is an important site of antiplatelet antibody production [40]. Some patients improve spontaneously in 1 to 2 years, so there is no rush to splenectomy [40]. If emergency treatment of ITP is required, then intravenous immunoglobulin (IVIG) and corticosteroids are the treatment of choice. If there is clinical bleeding, platelet transfusion or platelet transfusion in conjunction with continuous infusion IVIG may be administered [43].

In secondary immune thrombocytopenia treatment, the underlying cause of ITP may affect the treatment approach [40].

ITP secondary to Hepatitis C

The treatment is antiviral therapy. If therapy for ITP is required, then IVIG may be given [43]. Corticosteroids should be avoided as they may increase the HCV viral load [43]. Splenectomy and eltrombopag have also been used, and treatment should be coordinated with a hepatologist or infectious disease specialist [43].

ITP secondary to HIV

Highly active antiretroviral therapy (HAART) improves thrombocytopenia. Short term corticosteroids, IVIG, or WinRho may also be used [43]. Care in this group of patients should be coordinated with an infectious disease specialist [43].

ITP associated with H. Pylori

One should only test for *H. pylori*, via urea breath test, stool antigen test or endoscopic biopsy if the patient has indications for eradication therapy [43]. Eradication therapy only variably improves the platelet count in this condition [43].

Drug Induced Thrombocytopenia: Glycoprotein IIb/IIIa Antagonists

Abciximab (ReoPro), Tirofiban (Aggrastat), Eptifibatide (Integrilin)

The epidemiology of the thrombocytopenia is based upon the widespread use of GPIIb/IIIa antagonists in the treatment of acute coronary syndromes. The risk for thrombocytopenia is 0.3-1.6% with abciximab, 0.2- 0.4% with tirofiban, and up to 0.2% with eptifibatide [49].

Upon second exposure to the drug, there is a higher risk for the development of thrombocytopenia and to an even lower platelet count level [49]. The diagnosis of drug induced thrombocytopenia associated with the GPIIb/IIIa inhibitor drugs may be difficult because there has also been a pseudothrombocytopenia associated with their use, even in the setting of citrated blood [3]. As such, it is critical to look at the peripheral smear to exclude platelet clumps [3].

The clinical presentation here is unique to the GPIIb/IIIa inhibitors because the thrombocytopenia develops in a short time frame, within the first 24 hours of exposure. Platelets can drop to less than 20,000/mm^3 and there is an increased risk for bleeding [49]. The clinical symptoms include ecchymosis, petechial hemorrhages and wet purpura, manifested as blood blisters in the mouth. Wet purpura is a sign for increased risk of fatal intracranial bleeding. The peripheral smear findings are important here to confirm a low platelet count and the absence of platelet clumping [3].

The pathophysiology of the thrombocytopenia caused by GPIIb/IIIa antagonists is felt to be an immune mediated thrombocytopenia [49]. Since the GPIIb/IIIa inhibitors lower platelet count within 1 to 2 days, it has been suggested that there are pre-existing antibodies that recognize neoepitopes when fiban binds to it, and this contributes to the rapid time course for the platelet count drop [8].

There is a clearing of platelets with antibodies specific to GPIIb/IIIa and eptifibatide [49]. For eptifibatide, the antiplatelet drug-dependent antibodies work against the megakaryocytes [7, 49].

Abciximab blocks platelet fibrinogen interaction. One percent of patients treated the first time and as many as ten percent of patients treated the second time develop acute thrombocytopenia within a few hours of the infusion [8]. There has been described a delayed thrombocytopenia, occurring 5 to 8 days after the initial 24-48 hour exposure to the drug. This delayed thrombocytopenia is caused by newly generated antibodies that recognize abciximab coated platelets [8]. Abciximab coated platelets remain in the circulation up to 10 to 14 days after treatment [8].

The treatment of choice here is to discontinue the drug. If one needs to support the thrombocytopenia, it should be done with platelet transfusion, especially in the setting of wet purpura or active bleeding. Fatal intracranial hemorrhage and pulmonary hemorrhage has been known to occur [8, 49]. Upon stopping the GPIIb/IIIa inhibitor, platelets usually normalize within 3 days. Occasionally, the thrombocytopenia can last longer with severe hemorrhage as already described in this chapter [49].

Part 4: Causes of Thrombocytopenia during Pregnancy

Spurious
Gestational
ITP
Preeclampsia and HELLP
TTP/HUS
HIT
Acute fatty liver of pregnancy
DIC
Antiphospholipid syndrome (APS)

Thrombocytopenia is a common problem during pregnancy with many potential etiologies as the cause. The problem can frequently be asymptomatic but can also progress to a severe disorder such as in preeclampsia [50-52].

Normal platelet counts are between 150,000/mm^3 and 400,000/mm^3. But a lower than normal platelet count during pregnancy would not be unheard of [53, 54].

Spurious

This is a problem not only seen in pregnancy and is felt to be due to EDTA-induced aggregation of platelets. The way to properly diagnose this problem would be to repeat a platelet count in another diluent, such as citrate or heparin.

Gestational

This is sometimes referred to as the "Incidental Thrombocytopenia" of pregnancy. It is characterized by the quantitative abnormality generally being mild and without symptoms as well as having no prior history of non-pregnancy related thrombocytopenia. It tends to occur in the later stages of pregnancy and is usually cured after delivery of the baby [55]. The platelet counts are usually between 70,000/mm^3 and 130,000/mm^3 [50]. Studies have shown that many of these patients develop antibodies which are difficult to distinguish from those seen in ITP [56, 57]. The most important things to consider in the differential diagnosis are ITP, preeclampsia and DIC.

The management is usually similar to normal obstetric patients. Consideration for the use of epidural or spinal anesthesia needs to be given when the platelet count is somewhere between 50,000/mm^3 and 80,000/mm^3 [58]. Usually, the natural course is for the platelet count to recover from gestational thrombocytopenia, but the mother is felt to be at risk for thrombocytopenia with subsequent pregnancies [59].

ITP

The subject of ITP is discussed in this book chapter as well as in another entire book chapter. The incidence of ITP in pregnancy has been reported to be anywhere from 1 in 1,000 to 1 in 10,000 [60-62]. The diagnosis is frequently indistinguishable from gestational thrombocytopenia. The most significant concern clinically is the risk for maternal hemorrhage. Generally platelet transfusion is indicated for a platelet count of less than 30,000/mm^3 or in the presence of significant bleeding with a platelet count of less than 50,000/mm^3 [6, 43]. In one retrospective study, 31 percent of the women required a platelet transfusion [60].

Glucocorticoids may have a slight advantage over IVIG in pregnancy with respect to maintaining the platelet count for a longer period of time [43]. Splenectomy, rituximab and the thrombopoietin antagonists should be avoided during pregnancy [43].

Similar concerns for the use of epidural and spinal anesthesia are relevant and the risk and benefits need to be discussed in a multidisciplinary approach with the obstetrician, anesthesiologist and the patient.

As a separate issue but not for discussion here, are the neonatal risks of bleeding associated with maternal ITP, the most severe manifestation of which is that of a neonatal intracranial hemorrhage, which is quite rare.

Preeclampsia and HELLP

Preeclampsia is a syndrome that is uniquely associated with pregnancy. Clinically, this usually manifests itself with hypertension (levels can be as low as a systolic BP of 140-150 mm Hg) and proteinuria. This disorder is most likely to be seen in the third trimester, but can also occur in the postpartum period [63]. When seizures occur, the diagnosis of eclampsia is made. Thrombocytopenia is well described as a complication of preeclampsia, with an incidence reported to be as high as 15 percent with the degree of thrombocytopenia being severe in about 5 percent of those cases [64]. When the thrombocytopenia is severe, one must also consider the diagnosis of HELLP syndrome (**H**emolysis, **E**levated **L**iver enzymes and **L**ow **P**latelets) or DIC [65, 66]. It is sometimes difficult to distinguish HELLP from disorders discussed already in this chapter such as TTP and HUS [66, 67].

In HELLP, there is a common physical examination finding of pain or tenderness in the right upper quadrant, but this is also easily confused with acute fatty liver of pregnancy. However, unless there is another reason for thrombocytopenia present, acute fatty liver of pregnancy rarely gives the patient thrombocytopenia in and of itself. Preeclampsia usually resolves relatively quickly after delivery or soon thereafter. One of the keys that one may be dealing with TTP or HUS for example is that severe neurologic deficits have developed and that the platelet disturbance persists for more than a few days postpartum.

The preferred treatment of choice for preeclampsia, eclampsia and HELLP is delivery of the fetus. If the hematologic and neurologic manifestations fail to resolve within 72 hours after delivery, serious consideration must be given to treat as a TTP or HUS patient.

TTP and HUS

A significant relationship between both TTP and HUS and pregnancy has been established. Reports regarding the incidence of TTP and HUS in pregnant patients in various series have been between 10 and 25 percent [68-70]. If a patient had been diagnosed with TTP or HUS prior to their pregnancy, they are at an increased risk for a relapse during their subsequent pregnancies [67, 71, 72]. The Oklahoma registry reports that about 12 percent of patients in their data base developed TTP or HUS with a subsequent pregnancy [73].

One study suggested that the majority of TTP and HUS cases that occur during pregnancy happen in the 2nd and 3rd trimester [67].

Once the diagnosis is established or if there is a high suspicion, treatment remains the same as it is in the non-pregnant patient, which is plasma exchange. Although there is no data to support delivery of the fetus, this is advocated by some maternal-fetal medicine experts.

HIT

Heparin induced thrombocytopenia is discussed in Part 1 of this chapter. It is infrequently seen as a cause of thrombocytopenia in pregnancy but must remain in the differential diagnosis of thrombocytopenia that develops in the peripartum or postpartum period.

Acute Fatty Liver of Pregnancy

While thrombocytopenia is not a prominent feature of this disorder, one of the laboratory manifestations seen may be the presence of thrombocytopenia with or without concomitant DIC. Here the mechanism of the platelet disturbance may be due to decreased levels of antithrombin III [74].

DIC

Disseminated intravascular coagulopathy in pregnancy is a disorder that has been reported in anywhere from 9.2 to 12.5 for every 10,000 maternal deliveries and is the cause of about 25 percent of all maternal deaths [75, 76]. There are unique complications of pregnancy that predispose a mother to developing DIC. These include problems such as uterine hemorrhage due to uterine rupture, placenta previa, and placenta accreta or from uterine atony post-delivery; as well as preeclampsia-eclampsia, HELLP syndrome, amniotic fluid embolism, septic abortion and placental abruption. It is also important not to forget the other common causes of DIC that are unrelated specifically to pregnancy such as sepsis or trauma for example.

There are well known changes to the coagulation system that occur during pregnancy essentially to assure that excessive bleeding or hemorrhage will not complicate the delivery process. The pathophysiology of various pregnancy related causes of DIC has been described in another section of this chapter and we will not take the time to discuss each one individually for the purpose of this book chapter [77]. Clinically during pregnancy, we are most concerned about severe bleeding, the development of either hemorrhagic or distributive shock and the possibility of progressing to multiorgan dysfunction syndrome (MODS).

The treatment should mostly be focused on what has triggered the development of DIC and to reverse or fix the underlying disturbance. Management of this condition in pregnancy also includes a multidisciplinary approach to management that includes the obstetrician (maternal-fetal medicine expert), the anesthesiologist, the neonatologist, the blood bank staff and possibly the critical care team. Having appropriate intravenous access for the patient is crucial to proper management.

The patient may require a variety of different blood products including packed RBCs, platelets, fresh frozen plasma (FFP) and cryoprecipitate. Delivery of the fetus should be the focus and preparation should be in place for vaginal delivery or caesarian section.

Antiphospholipid Syndrome (APS)

There is the possibility of developing thrombocytopenia in the APS. This has been discussed in this chapter previously. As it relates to pregnancy, thrombocytopenia in the presence of APS could lead to early fetal loss or fetal demise, or late complications such as placental insufficiency or preeclampsia.

References

[1] Hunt, B. J. Bleeding and coagulopathies in critical care. *N. Eng. J. Med.* 2014; 370(9): 847-859.

[2] *ASH-SAP American Society of Hematology Self-Assessment Program. Textbook.* 5th Edition. Washington, DC 2013.

[3] Greinacher, A., Selleng, K. Thrombocytopenia in the Intensive Care Unit Patient. Hematology 2010. *American Society of Hematology Education Program Book.* 135-143.

[4] Lichtman, M., Beutler, E., et al. *Williams Manual of Hematology Sixth Edition.* McGraw-Hill Medical Publishing Division. New York. 2003.

[5] Naik, U. P. Bacteria exploit platelets. *Blood.* 2014; 123(20):3067-3068.

[6] Arman, M., Krauel, K., et al. Amplification of bacteria-induced platelet activation is triggered by FcyRIIA, integrin aIIbβ3, and platelet factor 4. *Blood.* 2014; 123(20): 3166-3174.

[7] Perdomo, J., Yan, F., et al. Quinine-induced thrombocytopenia: drug-dependent GP1b/IX antibodies inhibit megakaryocyte and proplatelet production in vitro. *Blood.* 2011;117(22):5975-5986.

[8] Aster, R. H., Bougie, D. W. Current concepts drug-induced immune thrombocytopenia. *N. Eng. J. Med.* 2007;357(6):580-587.

[9] Bautista, M. A., Stevens, W. T., et al. Hypersensitivity reaction and acute immune-mediated thrombocytopenia from oxaliplatin: two case reports and a review of the literature. *J. Hematol. Oncol.* 2010; 3:12.

[10] Mason, J. M., Rees, G. J. G. Oxaliplatin-induced acute thrombocytopenia. *Journal of Oncology Pharmacy Practice.* 2010;17(4):433-435.

[11] Cuker, A., Gimotty, P. A., et al. Predictive value of the 4Ts scoring system for heparin-induced thrombocytopenia: a systematic review and meta-analysis. *Blood.* 2012; 120 (20):4160-4167.

[12] Warkentin, T. E. How I Diagnose and Manage HIT. *Hematology Am. Soc. Hematol. Educ. Program.* 2011;2011:143-9.

[13] Potschke, C., Selleng, S., et al. Heparin-induced thrombocytopenia: further evidence for a unique immune response. *Blood.* 2012;120:4238-4245.

[14] Cuker, A., Cines, D. B. How I treat heparin-induced thrombocytopenia. *Blood.* 2012; 119(10):2209-2218.

[15] Murphy, G. S., Marymont, J. H. Alternative anticoagulation management strategies for the patient with Heparin-Induced Thrombocytopenia undergoing cardiac surgery. *Journal of Cardiothoracic and Vascular Anesthesia.* 2007; 21(1):113-126.

[16] Rice, L., Attisha, W., et al. Delayed-Onset Heparin-Induced Thrombocytopenia. *Ann. Int. Med.* 2002;136(3):210-215.

[17] Warkentin, T. E., Greinacher, A. Heparin-Induced Thrombocytopenia and Cardiac Surgery. *Ann. Thorac. Surg.* 2003;76:2121-2131.

[18] Wartenkin, T. E., Sheppard, J. I. Serological investigation of patients with a previous history of heparin-induced thrombocytopenia who are re-exposed to heparin. *Blood.* 2014; Feb. 10; (http://dx.doi.org/10.1182/blood-2013-10-533083).

[19] Allen, D. L., Samol, J., et al. Survey of the use and clinical effectiveness of HPA-1a/5b-negative platelet concentrates in proven or suspected platelet alloimmunization. *Transfusion Medicine*. 2004;14(6):409-417.

[20] Christie, D. J., Pulkrabek, S., et al. Posttransfusion purpura due to an alloantibody reactive with Glycoprotein Ia/IIa (Anti-HPA-5b). *Blood*. 1991; 77(12): 2785-2789.

[21] Lichtman, M., Beutler, E., Kipps, T. J., et al. *Williams Hematology Seventh Edition*. McGraw-Hill Companies, Inc. 2006.

[22] Fuchs, T. A., Kremer Hovinga, J. A., et al. Circulating DNA and myeloperoxidase indicate disease activity in patients with thrombotic microangiopathies. *Blood*. 2012; 120:1157-1164.

[23] Greinacher, A., Friesecke, S., et al. Treatment of severe neurological deficits with IgG depletion through immunoadsorption in patients with Escherichia coli O104:H4-associated haemolytic uraemic syndrome: a prospective trial. *The Lancet*. 378:1166-1173.

[24] George, J. N. How I treat patients with thrombotic thrombocytopenic purpura: 2010. *Blood*. 2010; 116(2):4060-4069.

[25] Cataland, S. R., Wu, H. M. How I treat: the clinical differentiation and initial treatment of adult patients with atypical hemolytic ureic syndrome. *Blood*. 2014; 123(16):2478-2484.

[26] Nackos, E., DeSancho, M. Anemia and thrombocytopenia: diagnosis from the blood smear. *Blood*. 2014; 123(12):1783.

[27] Dlevaeye, M., Noris, M., et al. Thrombomodulin mutations in atypical hemolytic-uremic syndrome. *N. Eng. J. Med*. 2009; 361(4):345-357.

[28] Scully, M., Hunt, B. J., et al. Guidelines on the diagnosis and management of thrombotic thrombocytopenic purpura and other thrombotic microangiopathies. *British Journal of Haematology*. 2012; 158:323-335.

[29] Scully, M., McDonald, V., et al. A phase 2 study of the safety and efficacy of rituximab with plasma exchange in acute acquired thrombotic thrombocytopenic purpura. *Blood*. 2011; 118:1746-1753.

[30] Deford, C., Reese, J. A., et al. Multiple major morbidities and increased mortality during long-term follow-up after recovery from thrombotic thrombocytopenic purpura. *Blood*. 2013 Sep. 19;122(12):2023-9; quiz 2142. doi: 10.1182/blood-2013-04-496752. Epub. 2013 Jul. 9.

[31] Cornellas-Kirkerup, L., Hernandez-Molina, G., et al. Antiphospholipid-associated thrombocytopenia or autoimmune hemolytic anemia in patients with or without definite primary antiphospholipid syndrome according to the Sapporo revised classification criteria: a 6-year follow-up study. *Blood*. 2010; 116 3-58-3063.

[32] Ortona, E., Capozzi, A., et al. Vimentin/cardiolipin complex as a new antigenic target of the antiphospholipid syndrome. *Blood*. 2010; 116:2960-2967.

[33] Clark, C. A., Davidovits, J., et al. The lupus anticoagulant results from 2257 patients attending a high-risk pregnancy clinic. *Blood*. 2013; 122:341-347.

[34] Shanafelt, T. D., Madueme, H. L., et al. Rituximab for immune cytopenia in adults: Idiopathic Thrombocytopenic Purpura, Autoimmune Hemolytic Anemia, and Evans Syndrome. *Mayo Clinic Proceedings*. 2003; 78:1340-1346.

[35] Branchford, B. R., DiPaola, J. Making a diagnosis of VWD. *Hematology Am. Soc. Hematol. Educ. Program.* 2012;2012:161-7. doi: 10.1182/asheducation-2012.1.161. Review.
[36] Afdhal, N. H., Giannini, E. G., et al. Eltrombopag before procedures in patients with cirrhosis and thrombocytopenia. *N. Eng. J. Med.* 2012; 367(7):716-724.
[37] Anderson, S. C., Poulsen, K. B. *Anderson's Atlas of Hematology*. 2003. Lippincott Williams and Wilkins.
[38] McHutchison, J. G., Dusheiko, G. Eltrombopag for thrombocytopenia in patients with cirrhosis associated with hepatitis C. *N. Eng. J. Med.* 2007; 357(22):2227-2236.
[39] Will, B., Kawahara, M., et al. Effect of the nonpeptide thrombopoietin receptor agonist Eltrombopag on bone marrow cells from patients with acute myeloid leukemia and myelodysplastic syndrome. *Blood.* 2009; 114(18): 3899-3908.
[40] Ghanima, W., Godeau, B., et al. How I treat immune thrombocytopenia: the choice between splenectomy or a medical therapy as a second-line treatment. *Blood.* 2012; 120 (5) 960-969.
[41] Mir, M. A. Dysarthria and thrombocytopenia after tick bite. *Blood.* 2013; 122(15):2538.
[42] Grimaldi-Bensouda, L., Michel, M., et al. A case-control study to assess the risk of immune thrombocytopenia associated with vaccines. *Blood.* 2012; 120(25): 4938-4944.
[43] Neunert, C., Lim, W., et al. The American Society of Hematology 2011 evidence-based practice guideline for immune thrombocytopenia. *Blood.* 2011; 117(16):4190-4207.
[44] Hammerschmidt, D. E. Szechwan Purpura. *N. Eng. J. Med.* 1980; 302(21):1191-1193.
[45] Arnason, J. E., Campigotto, F., et al. Abnormalities in IgA and IgM are associated with treatment-resistant ITP. *Blood.* 2012; 119(21):5016-5020.
[46] Godeau, B., Chevret, S., et al. Intravenous immunoglobulin or high-dose methylprednisolone, with or without oral prednisone, for adults with untreated severe autoimmune thrombocytopenic purpura: a randomized, multicentre trial. *The Lancet.* 2002: 359:23-29.
[47] Gudbrandsdottir, S., Birgens, H. S., et al. Rituximab and dexamethasone vs dexamethasone monotherapy in newly diagnosed patients with primary immune thrombocytopenia. *Blood.* 2013; 121(11):1976-1981.
[48] Kuter, D. J., Mufti, G. J., et al. Evaluation of bone marrow reticulin formation in chronic immune thrombocytopenia patients treated with romiplostim. *Blood.* 2009; 114 (18):33748-3756.
[49] Greinacher, A., Fueril, B., et al. Megakaryocyte impairment by eptifibatide-induced antibodies causes prolonged thrombocytopenia. *Blood.* 2009; 114(6): 1250-1253.
[50] Burrows, R. F., Kelton, J. G. Fetal thrombocytopenia and its relation to maternal thrombocytopenia. *N. Engl. J. Med.* 1993;329(20):1463.
[51] Saftlas, A. F., Olson, D. R., Franks, A. L., Atrash, H. K., Pokras, R. Epidemiology of preeclampsia and eclampsia in the United States, 1979-1986. *Am. J. Obstet. Gynecol.* 1990;163(2):460.
[52] Myers, B. Diagnosis and management of maternal thrombocytopenia in pregnancy. *Br. J. Haematol.* 2012;158(1) 3.
[53] Matthews, J. H., Benjamin, S., Gill, D. S., Smith, N. A. Pregnancy-associated thrombocytopenia: definition, incidence and natural history. *Acta Haematol.* 1990;84 (1):24.

[54] Boehlen, F., Hohlfeld, P., Extermann, P., Perneger, T. V., de Moerloose, P. Platelet count at term pregnancy: a reappraisal of the threshold. *Obstet. Gynecol.* 2000;95(1):29.
[55] George, J. N., Woolf, S. H., Raskob, G. E., Wasser, J. S., Aledort, L. M., Ballem, P. J., Blanchette, V. S., Bussel, J. B., Cines, D. B., Kelton, J. G., Lichtin, A. E., McMillan, R., Okerbloom, J. A., Regan, D. H., Warrier, I. Idiopathic thrombocytopenic purpura: a practice guideline developed by explicit methods for the American Society of Hematology. *Blood.* 1996;88(1):3.
[56] Lescale, K. B., Eddleman, K. A., Cines, D. B., Samuels, P., Lesser, M. L., McFarland, J. G., Bussel, J. B. Antiplatelet antibody testing in thrombocytopenic pregnant women. *Am. J. Obstet. Gynecol.* 1996;174(3):1014.
[57] Ajzenberg, N., Dreyfus, M., Kaplan, C., Yvart, J., Weill, B., Tchernia, G. Pregnancy-associated thrombocytopenia revisited: assessment and follow-up of 50 cases. *Blood.* 1998;92(12):4573.
[58] Shalev, O., Anteby, E. Epidural anesthesia can be safely performed in gestational thrombocytopenia
[59] Anteby, E., Shalev, O. Clinical relevance
[60] Burrows, R. F., Kelton, J. G. Pregnancy in patients with idiopathic.
[61] Webert, K. E., Mittal, R., Sigouin, C., et al. A retrospective 11-year analysis of obstetric patients with idiopathic
[62] Gill, K. K., Kelton, J. G. Management of idiopathic
[63] Cunningham, F. G., Lindheimer, M. D. Hypertension in pregnancy. *N. Engl. J. Med.* 1992; 326:927.
[64] Burrows, R. F., Kelton, J. G. Fetal thrombocytopenia
[65] Sibai, B. M., Ramadan
[66] Weiner, C. P. Thrombotic microangiopathy in pregnancy
[67] Martin, J. N. Jr, Bailey, A. P., Rehberg, J. F., et al. Thrombotic thrombocytopenic purpura
[68] Amorosi, E. L., Ultmann, J. E. Thrombotic thrombocytopenic purpura
[69] Ezra, Y., Rose, M., Eldor, A. Therapy and prevention
[70] George, J. N. The association of pregnancy
[71] Dashe, J. S., Ramin, S. M., Cunningham, F. G. The long-term consequences of thrombotic microangiopathy (thrombotic thrombocytopenic purpura
[72] Mokrzycki, M. H., Rickles, F. R., Kaplan, A. A., Kohn, O. F. Thrombotic thrombocytopenic purpura
[73] Vesely, S. K., Li, X., McMinn, J. R., et al. Pregnancy outcomes after recovery
[74] Castro, M. A., Goodwin, T. M., Shaw, K. J., et al. Disseminated intravascular coagulation and antithrombin III depression
[75] Callaghan, W. M., Creanga, A. A., Kuklina, E. V. Severe maternal morbidity
[76] Thachil, J., Toh, C. H. Disseminated intravascular coagulation in obstetric disorders and its acute haematological management
[77] Levi, M. Disseminated intravascular coagulation (DIC) in pregnancy

In: Thrombocytopenia
Editor: Mckenzie G. Bell

ISBN: 978-1-63321-713-3

Chapter 3

New Treatment for ITP for a Subset of Patients

***Barry Bockow, MD, FACP*[1,2*] *and Tamara B. Kaplan, MD*[3]**
[1]Arthritis Northwest, Seattle, WA
[2]University of Washington School of Medicine, Seattle, WA
[3]Massachusetts General Hospital/Brigham and Women's Hospital, Boston, MA

Abstract

Immune thrombocytopenic purpura (ITP) is an autoimmune disorder characterized by an immune response against the host's own platelets. The goal of treatment is to keep the platelet count above 30 $x10^9/L$ to prevent major internal organ bleeding. The initial therapy involves high dose steroids and or intravenous immunoglobulin IVIG. If unsuccessful, other immunosuppressant agents or biologic agents are used. Splenectomy also has been used with variable response. All of these therapies have considerable toxicity.

In the past we have identified a subset of patients who were refractory to treatment. These ITP patients had positive ANA's and were vitamin D deficient. Clinically they had SLE and Sjögren's syndrome overlap syndrome. Their response to high dose vitamin D replacement and hydroxychloroquine was dramatic. Their platelet counts normalized, but upon discontinuation of high dose vitamin D, platelet counts plummeted. With reinstitution of vitamin D, platelet counts were again restored. No untoward side effects were observed.

Recent research has shown that vitamin D deficiency is associated with increased cardiovascular risk, osteoporosis, cancer, diabetes type I in children, and autoimmune diseases such as multiple sclerosis and Crohn's disease. Previously we found an association between vitamin D deficiency and immune thrombocytopenia. There may also be synergism between vitamin D supplementation and hydroxychloroquine. Vitamin D has long been thought to play an immunomodulatory role. Specifically, 1,25(OH)2D3 seems to have two important functions: down regulation of over proliferative CD4+ cells and up regulation of T regulatory cells.

* Corresponding author: Barry Bockow, MD bockowmd@gmail.com.

Introduction

Immune Thrombocytopenic Purpura

Immune thrombocytopenic purpura (ITP) is thought to be an autoimmune disorder mediated by auto antibodies with no known etiology. Two mechanisms are involved in ITP: 1) accelerated platelet destruction, and 2) decreased platelet production by megakaryocytes in the bone marrow. In each individual various proportions of these 2 mechanisms are present. The variance of these mechanisms per individual patient dictates the treatment options. When no underlying cause of the thrombocytopenia is present it is called primary ITP.

Sometimes one can identify a secondary cause of ITP. This is important since one needs to treat the underlying cause. Some of these include *H. pylori*, hepatitis C, and lymphoproliferative disorders including non-Hodgkin's lymphoma, a myelodysplastic syndrome especially in elderly patients, chronic lymphocytic leukemia, Hodgkin's lymphoma, HIV, SLE (systemic lupus erythematosus) and other autoimmune diseases. Thrombocytopenia can also be caused by the antiphospholipid syndrome, autoimmune thyroid disease and immunodeficiency states including IgA deficiency. Drug-induced ITP is always an important consideration; drugs such as quinine, sulfonamides, and heparin are common causes of thrombocytopenia.

Treatment of ITP

There is currently no standard treatment for ITP. There are many therapeutic options, but each has considerable associated toxicities and variable efficacy [1, 2]. The usual and standard treatment involves high-dose prednisone [3]. This can be administered either orally or by IV. Recently, pulse dexamethasone therapy has been used by some groups. Intravenous immunoglobulin (IVIG) is a first-line treatment, however, the results are often transient and it is associated with numerous side effects including renal insufficiency and anaphylaxis. It is also very expensive. But, during the acute setting, especially in patients who are bleeding, it should be considered since it can raise the platelet count quickly. IV anti-Rho (D) is an alternative to IVIG [4]. However, it is not effective in Rh negative patients or in those who have undergone a splenectomy. Hemolysis is a rare complication to this therapy. Side effects include IV hemolysis, renal failure and disseminated intravascular coagulation (DIC).

Second-line therapies include a variety of chemotherapeutic agents, including Imuran, Cytoxan and cyclosporin A [1]. Other agents include CellCept and Rituxan [1]. Some of the toxicities associated with Rituxan include an infusion reaction and opportunistic infections, including progressive multifocal leukoencephalopathy .

Newer treatments include thrombopoietin receptor agonists (romiplostim [Nplate] and eltrombopag [Promacta]) that have been used in phase 3 studies of primary ITP to augment platelet production [5-7]. These agents increase platelet counts in both splenectomized and non-splenectomized patients. Some of the adverse effects include rebound thrombocytopenia, which occurs upon discontinuation of the drugs; bone marrow fibrosis, which occurs in less than 10% of treated patients; thrombosis, which occurs in approximately 5% of patients; progression to hematologic malignancies; and liver toxicity.

When treating secondary ITP related to HIV and hepatitis C [8], it is essential that one always treat the underlying cause/infection with antiviral agents. Splenectomy is effective in some cases but is usually not done in the first year because some cases do remit spontaneously. In addition, this procedure is associated with pulmonary hypertension and thrombosis as well as secondary infection with *H. influenzae* and other pathogens. After 10 years, two thirds of patients remain in remission after splenectomy [9, 10].

Diagnosis of ITP

A diagnosis of ITP is one of exclusion. The workup should include a peripheral blood smear. The red cell and white cell morphology is usually normal. One needs to exclude the presence of schistocytes and/or nucleated red blood cells, which would indicate a hemolytic anemia. Immunoglobulin levels should be checked. Additionally, antiphospholipid antibodies and ANA are measured, and the presence of HIV, hepatitis C, *H. pylori*, parvovirus and CMV is determined. Generally, testing for platelet antibodies is not recommended, and bone marrow examination is generally not necessary.

Vitamin D and Autoimmunity

Vitamin D Deficiency

Vitamin D deficiency is associated with many autoimmune diseases, including multiple sclerosis, SLE and type 1 diabetes [11]. In 2010, investigators analyzed serum vitamin D levels in SLE patients and found an inverse correlation between SLE severity and vitamin D concentration [12]. A recent study found SLE patients with higher vitamin D levels were less likely to develop serious complications from cardiovascular disease [13]. This pattern is also present in those with Crohn's disease [14].

Vitamin D Replacement Therapy

Vitamin D supplementation has been suggested as a possible co-treatment option for type 1 diabetes, SLE and Crohn's disease [15-18]. The Hopkins Cohort followed 1,000 patients from 2009 to 2011 with SLE who received vitamin D supplementation because of low levels < 40 ng/ml. They found a significant correlation between increased vitamin D levels and both a decreased risk of SLE severity and improved urine protein-creatinine ratio [15]. A meta-analysis of one cohort and four case-control studies investigating effects of vitamin D supplementation in infants on the development of type 1 diabetes found correlations between vitamin D and reduced diabetes risk [19].

Case Studies

Our group previously reported on two patients with severe ITP who failed conventional therapies but responded to Plaquenil (hydroxychloroquine) and high-dose vitamin D, which resulted in a marked increase in platelet counts [20]. Both patients were ANA+ and felt to have SLE as the cause of ITP. The two cases are described below.

Patient 1

Because of failure to respond to conventional therapy, the oncology service referred this patient to our clinic. They treated the patient with WinRho (IV Immune globulin, or IVIg) and high-dose prednisone due to an extremely low platelet count of 9,000/mm^3. The count transiently increased to 43,000/mm^3, suggesting prednisone treatment had little therapeutic effect. Upon referral to our clinic, we did a serological workup that revealed the presence of anti-SSA/Ro autoantibodies (SSA) and antinuclear antibodies (ANA), which suggested SLE and Sjögren's syndrome overlap as secondary causes for ITP.

To treat the ITP, we administered Plaquenil (200 mg twice a day), prednisone (15 mg/day) and high-dose vitamin D (50,000 IU once a week). This was initiated because of the borderline low vitamin D level of 34 ng/mL. In our experience with other autoimmune diseases we have found an enhanced therapeutic response to standard treatment when a patient's vitamin D increases to 40-50 ng/mL or above.

Two weeks post initial visit, the patient's platelet count slightly increased to 55,000/mm^3, but was still significantly under the normal value of >140,000/mm^3 (Figure 1A). To achieve an enhanced clinical benefit, vitamin D dosing was increased to 150,000 IU per week, prednisone was decreased to 10 mg/day and Plaquenil remained the same. On this new regimen, the platelet count increased (114,000/ mm^3) and vitamin D was then lowered to 50,000 IU twice a week, prednisone lowered to 5 mg/day, and as before Plaquenil was not altered.

Three months after the initial visit, the patient's platelet count had increased to 141,000/mm^3. Vitamin D, prednisone and Plaquenil remained the same. Because the patient's platelet count remained stable for approximately six months on this regimen and vitamin D levels were normal, high-dose vitamin D supplementation was discontinued. One month later, the patient's platelet count strikingly decreased by 100-fold to 18,000/mm^3 (Figure 1B). Responding to this life threatening drop, we immediately restarted vitamin D treatment (50,000 IU twice a week) and increased prednisone (30 mg/day). After three weeks, the platelet count increased to 91,000/mm^3. One month later the platelet count once again increased to normal levels and therefore prednisone treatment was reduced to 5 mg/day.

Four months later, the patient's platelet count reached 161,000/mm^3, and prednisone was discontinued. Six weeks after discontinuing prednisone, the platelet count continued to increase to 215,000/mm^3. Based on these results, we continued Plaquenil 200 mg twice a day and vitamin D 50,000 IU once a week. We did feel prednisone was not necessary for maintenance therapy.

Patient 2

The second patient was referred by the oncology service having failed conventional therapy. Like the first patient, the serology was positive for ANA and SSA and was diagnosed as having SLE and Sjögren's overlap with secondary ITP. It was noteworthy that the vitamin D level was severely depressed at 17 ng/mL and the platelet count was 8,000/mm^3. When treating secondary ITP it is essential to treat the underlying disease. We initiated Plaquenil 200 mg twice a day and continued prednisone at 40 mg/day, as prescribed earlier by the heme-oncology service. Vitamin D was dispensed at 50,000 IU once a week.

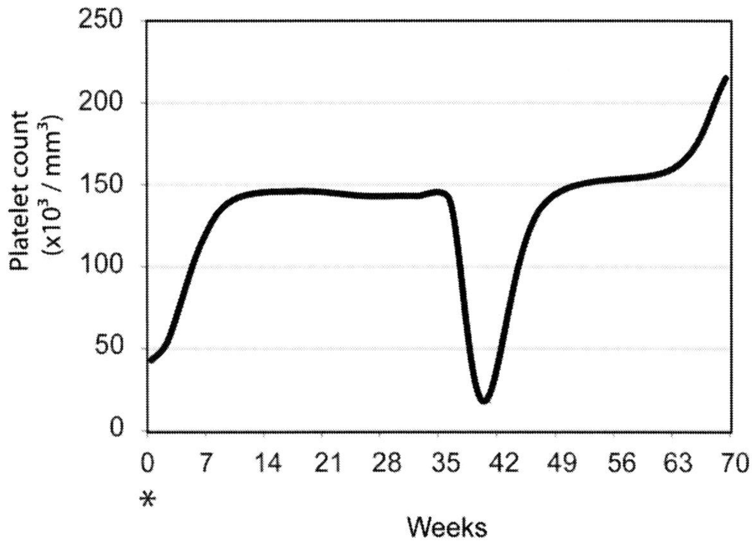

A

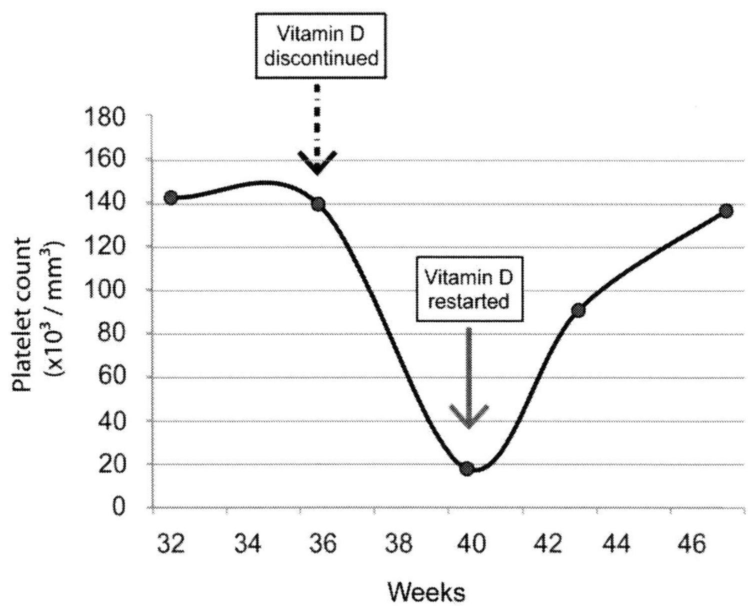

B

Figure 1. A. Platelet count levels over time. We measured Patient 1's platelet levels throughout the course of treatment.* denotes initiation of treatment. The x-axis depicts time in weeks; the y-axis depicts platelet count (x 10^3/mm^3). B. Platelet count in relation to vitamin D. Close-up of weeks 32-47 from part A. At the time of vitamin D discontinuation the platelet count was 140,000/mm^3 (black hashed arrow). After one month, the platelet count plummeted to 18,000/mm^3. In response to reinstitution of vitamin D therapy (grey arrow) the platelet count increased to 91,000/mm^3 after three weeks and then 137,000/mm^3 four weeks later. The x-axis depicts time in weeks; the y-axis depicts platelet count (x 10^3/mm^3).

One month later the platelet counts increased to 72,000/mm^3, and prednisone was tapered from 40 mg/day to 15 mg/day. Six weeks after initiation of treatment, the patient's platelet count had again increased (to 301,000/mm^3) and therefore prednisone was lowered to 7.5

mg/day. Six weeks weeks later the platelet count dropped to 89,000/mm^3 and therefore vitamin D was increased to 50,000 IU twice a week. With this dosage change, the patient was doing well and the platelet count had increased to 244,000/mm^3. Vitamin D levels reached almost 90 ng/mL; therefore prednisone was tapered to 5 mg and vitamin D supplementation remained at 50,000 IU twice week. After nine weeks on this dosage, platelet counts stabilized to approximately 190,000/mm^3 and remained stable at prednisone of 4 mg/day. The counts continued in this range for another 10 months.

Four-and-a-half years post-initial presentation the patient remained in remission and continued on a reduced dose of Plaquenil, namely 200 mg/day, prednisone 2 mg/day and vitamin D 50,000 units once a month.

Discussion

Autoimmune platelet depletion, such as with ITP, occurs when autoantibodies targeting glycoproteins found on the surface of platelets opsonize the cells, resulting in destruction by macrophages. Because these levels are regulated by both the production and clearance of platelets, a fine balance must exist. Ongoing destruction of platelets and an inadequate production of new platelets will foster disease.

It has been documented that patients with immune thrombocytopenia have high rates of mononuclear cell proliferation as well as lymphocytes that secrete greater amounts of IL-2 compared to controls [21]. Researchers have also shown that in these patients, depleting CD8$^+$ lymphocytes and complement did not reduce proliferation of mononuclear cells, which indicates that CD4$^+$ T helper cells may be responsible for the response. In addition, the number of T regulatory cells in patients with ITP is markedly reduced [22]. This suggests that stimulated CD4$^+$ T helper cells mediate antibody production and maturation of B cells, and may contribute to the eventual autoantibody response targeting these patients' platelets.

Activation of vitamin D receptors (VDRs) is known to alter immune cell transcriptional patterns, proliferation and differentiation through several intracellular pathways. Both CD4$^+$ and CD8$^+$ lymphocytes express VDRs, and thus it is reasonable to conclude that vitamin D (25(OH)2D3) may play a role in the regulation of the immune response [23]. A meta analysis of publications identifying VDR polymorphisms uncovered a significantly higher risk of the inflammatory bowel disease Crohn's from one polymorphism and a lower risk of ulcerative colitis due to a different mutation [24]. Genetic polymorphisms in these receptors also correlate with other autoimmune diseases including type 2 diabetes, multiple sclerosis and SLE [25-27]. It's also seen in breast and skin cancer [28, 29]. Interestingly, several of these studies identified differences within specific ethnic groups.

25(OH)2D3 may be a potent immunomodulator, and it may have potential therapeutic use in many autoimmune diseases [11]. In 1991, researchers found that the production of interleukin IL-6 and IL-2 in cell cultures were reduced by vitamin D [30]. It was postulated that vitamin D may inhibit the production and function of IL-6 and, therefore, regulate lymphocyte functions. Studies have shown that 25(OH)2D3 can inhibit the development of multiple sclerosis in the murine model [31,32]. Researchers suggest that CD4$^+$ T cells may be the target of immunosuppression and studies have found that 25(OH)2D3 can inhibit T-cell proliferation and activation [33].

A subset of helper T cells called TH17 cells have been found at sites of autoimmune inflammation and thus may be a main contributor to tissue destruction in patients suffering from such diseases [34]. Although the molecular mechanisms have not been fully elucidated, vitamin D has an inhibitory effect on these TH17 cells. In the murine model of scleroderma, topical administration with the vitamin D analog calcipotriol resulted in an increase in the Th2-mediated pro-fibrotic pathway, but the treatment actually had a net anti-fibrotic effect [35]. This study suggests that calcipotriol could be a potential therapeutic for treating fibrotic disease in humans.

Vitamin D stimulates transforming growth factor (TGFβ-1) and IL-4 production, which in turn may suppress inflammatory T-cell activity [36, 37]. TGFβ-1 may help direct T-cell differentiation and promote the production of T regulatory cells via the Foxp3 transcription regulatory pathway resulting in the observed immunosuppression [38]. In fact, TGFβ-1 is able to promote T-cell differentiation from non-suppressor $CD4^+$ T cells simply through Foxp3 induction [39]. These T regulatory cells help suppress the immune response and thus maintain immune system homeostasis and tolerance to self -antigens. Recently, it was shown that vitamin D treatment in addition to calcitriol transiently increased $Foxp3^+$ T cells and reduced the number of $CD4^+$ T cells in the spleens and CNS of mice with experimental autoimmune encephalomyelitis, the murine model for multiple sclerosis [40]. Cholecalciferol has been shown to increase the number of regulatory T cells when given in combination with insulin to those with new-onset type 1 diabetes [41].

Although the number of T regulatory cells in ITP patients is significantly reduced, research has also shown that it is possible to generate T regulatory cells in vitro by pharmacologically manipulating the dendritic cells with glucocorticoid and vitamin D [42]. Drug-induced effects on dendritic cells included induction of IL-10-secreting regulatory T cells, attenuation of IL-2 and interferon gamma secretion, prevention of T cell IL-4 secretion, and suppression of antigen-specific primary T-cell proliferation [43].

Overall, vitamin D seems to have two important immunomodulatory functions: down-regulation of over proliferative $CD4^+$ cells and concurrent up-regulation of T regulatory cells. Together, these effects may have the potential to reduce the autoantibody response and may potentially explain the restoration of platelet levels upon treatment of high-dose vitamin D in patients who had autoimmune thrombocytopenia.

Conclusion

We recommend that vitamin D levels be obtained on all patients who are thrombocytopenic; the high prevalence of vitamin D deficiency in the United States of America makes this particularly crucial. If vitamin D levels are less than 30 ng/Ml, we recommend the patient receive aggressive replacement with vitamin D supplementation at high doses. This is particularly relevant in a patient with secondary ITP who has an underlying autoimmune disease, such as SLE.

In our experience the therapeutic dose varies between 50,000 and 100,000 IU/week depending on the platelet count. This dose should be maintained for many months if the renal function remains normal. Additionally, it is recommended to monitor their serum calcium, phosphate, parathyroid hormone and creatinine levels. When the platelet count stabilizes, in some patients, vitamin D supplementation may need to be maintained indefinitely. We also suggest the addition of Plaquenil 200 mg twice a day, especially if the patient is ANA positive and/or there is a clinical suggestion of Sjögren's syndrome or SLE. We believe there is a synergistic effect of Plaquenil and high dose vitamin D. The mechanism of this interaction needs to be further defined. Additionally, it is important that investigators explore this further to confirm our findings and consider this regimen in the unique subset of patients who are ANA positive and vitamin D deficient, and have SLE. It is noteworthy that this treatment protocol is safe, effective and extremely inexpensive. Current treatments of ITP can be variable, have considerable side effects and are very costly.

References

[1] Provan D, Stasi R, Newland AC, Blanchette VS, Bolton-Maggs P, Bussel JB, Chong BH, Cines DB, Gernsheimer TB, Godeau B, Grainger J, Greer I, Hunt BJ, Imbach PA, Lyons G, McMillan R, Rodeghiero F, Sanz MA, Tarantino M, Watson S, Young J, Kuter DJ. International consensus report on the investigation and management of primary immune thrombocytopenia. *Blood*. 2010 Jan 14;115(2):168-86.

[2] Bromberg ME. Immune thrombocytopenic purpura—the changing therapeutic landscape. *N. Engl. J. Med.* 2006; 355:1643–1645.

[3] Cheng Y, Wong RS, Soo YO, et al. Initial treatment of immune thrombocytopenic purpura with high-dose dexamethasone. *N. Engl. J. Med.* 2003; 349:831–836.

[4] Scaradavou A, Woo B, Woloski BM, et al. Intravenous anti-D treatment of immune thrombocytopenic purpura: experience in 272 patients. *Blood* 1997; 89:2689–2700.

[5] Kuter DJ, Bussel JB, Lyons RM, et al. Efficacy of romiplostiminpatients with chronic immune thrombocytopenic purpura: a double-blind randomised controlled trial. *Lancet* 2008; 371:395-403.

[6] Gernsheimer TB, George JN, Aledort LM, et al. Evaluation of bleeding and thrombotic events during long-term use of romiplostim in patients with chronic immune thrombocytopenia (ITP). *J. Thromb. Haemost* 2010; 8:1372–1382.

[7] Cheng G, Saleh MN, Marcher C, et al. Eltrombopag for management of chronic immune thrombocytopenia (RAISE): a 6-month, randomised, phase 3 study. *Lancet* 2011 Jan 29;377(9763):393-402.

[8] Rajan SK, Espina BM, Liebman HA. Hepatitis Cvirus-related thrombocytopenia: clinical and laboratory characteristics compared with chronic immune thrombocytopenic purpura. *Br. J. Haematol.* 2005;129:818–824.

[9] Schwartz J, Leber MD, Gillis S, Giunta A, Eldor A, Bussel JB. Longterm follow-up after splenectomy performed for immune thrombocytopenic purpura (ITP). *Am. J. Hematol.* 2003;72:94–98.

[10] Kojouri K, Vesely SK, Terrell DR, George JN. Splenectomy for adult patients with idiopathic thrombocytopenic purpura: a systematic review to assess long-term platelet count responses, prediction of response, and surgical complications. *Blood* 2004;104:2623–2634.

[11] Yang CY, Leung PS, Adamopoulos IE, Gershwin ME. The implication of vitamin D and autoimmunity: a comprehensive review. *Clin. Rev. Allergy Immunol.* 2013 Oct;45(2):217-264.

[12] Amital H, Szekanecz Z, Szucs G, Dankó K, Nagy E, Csépány T, et al. Serum concentrations of 25-OH vitamin D in patients with systemic lupus erythematosus (SLE) are inversely related to disease activity: is it time to routinely supplement patients with SLE with vitamin D? *Annals of the rheumatic diseases*. 2010;69:1155–7.

[13] Lertratanakul A, Wu P, Dyer A, Urowitz M, Gladman D, Fortin P, Bae SC, Gordon C, Clarke A, Bernatsky S, Hanly JG, Isenberg D, Rahman A, Merrill J, Wallace DJ, Ginzler E, Khamashta M, Bruce I, Nived O, Sturfelt G, Steinsson K, Manzi S, Dooley MA, Kalunian K, Petri M, Aranow C, Font J, van Vollenhoven R, Stoll T,Ramsey-Goldman R. 25-Hydroxyvitamin D and cardiovascular disease in patients with systemic lupus erythematosus: Data from a large international inception cohort. *Arthritis Care Res. (Hoboken)*. 2014 Jan 27. [Epub ahead of print].

[14] Ham M, Longhi MS, Lahiff C, Cheifetz A, Robson S, Moss AC. Vitamin D levels in adults with Crohn's disease are responsive to disease activity and treatment. *Inflamm Bowel. Dis.* 2014 May;20(5):856-60.

[15] Petri M, Bello KJ, Fang H, Magder LS. Vitamin D in SLE: Modest association with disease activity and urine protein/creatinine ratio. *Arthritis rheum.*2013 Jul;65(7): 1865-71.

[16] Chakhtoura M, Azar ST. The role of vitamin d deficiency in the incidence, progression, and complications of type 1 diabetes mellitus. *Int. J. Endocrinol.* 2013;2013:148673.

[17] Wingate KE, Jacobson K, Issenman R, Carroll M, Barker C, Israel D, Brill H, Weiler H, Barr SI, Li W, Lyon MR, Green TJ. 25-Hydroxyvitamin D concentrations in children with Crohn's disease supplemented with either 2000 or 400 IU daily for 6 months: a randomized controlled study. *.J. Pediatr.* 2014 Apr;164(4):860-5.

[18] Mok CC. Vitamin D and systemic lupus erythematosus: an update. *Expert Rev Clin Immunol.* 2013 May;9(5):453-63.

[19] Zipitis CS, Akobeng AK. Vitamin D supplementation in early childhood and risk of type 1 diabetes: a systematic review and meta-analysis. *Arch. Dis. Child.* 2008 Jun;93(6):512-7.

[20] Bockow B, Kaplan TB. Refractory immune thrombocytopenia successfully treated with high-dose vitamin D supplementation and hydroxychloroquine: two case reports. *J. Med. Case Rep.* 2013 Apr 4;7(1):91.

[21] Andersson J: Cytokines in idiopathic thrombocytopenic purpura (ITP). *Acta Paediatr* Suppl 1998, 424:61-64.

[22] Semple JW, Freedman J. Increased antiplatelet T helper lymphocyte reactivity in patients with autoimmune thrombocytopenia. *Blood* 1991, 78(10):2619-2625.

[23] Veldman CM, Cantorna MT, DeLuca HF: Expression of 1,25-dihydroxyvitamin D(3) receptor in the immune system. *Arch. Biochem. Biophys.* 2000;374(2):334-338.

[24] Wang L, Wang ZT, Hu JJ, Fan R, Zhou J, Zhong J. Polymorphisms of the vitamin D receptor gene and the risk of inflammatory bowel disease: a meta-analysis. *Genet. Mol. Res.* 2014 Apr 8;13(2):2598-610.

[25] Al-Daghri NM, Al-Attas OS, Alkharfy KM, Khan N, Mohammed AK, Vinodson B, Ansari MG, Alenad A, Alokail MS.Association of VDR-gene variants with factors

related to the metabolic syndrome, type 2 diabetes and vitamin D deficiency. *Gene.* 2014 Jun 1;542(2):129-33.

[26] Harandi AA, Harandi AA, Pakdaman H, Sahraian MA. Vitamin D and multiple sclerosis. *Iran J. Neurol.* 2014;13(1):1-6.

[27] Zhou TB, Jiang ZP, Lin ZJ, Su N. Association of vitamin D receptor gene polymorphism with the risk of systemic lupus erythematosus. *J. Recept. Signal Transduct Res.* 2014 May 22:1-7. [Epub ahead of print]

[28] Zhang K, Song L. Association between Vitamin D Receptor Gene Polymorphisms and Breast Cancer Risk: A Meta-Analysis of 39 Studies. *PLoS One.* 2014 Apr 25;9(4):e96125.

[29] Zhao XZ, Yang BH, Yu GH, Liu SZ, Yuan ZY. Polymorphisms in the vitamin D receptor (VDR) genes and skin cancer risk in European population: a meta-analysis. *Arch. Dermatol. Res.* 2014 Apr 28. [Epub ahead of print]

[30] Muller K, Diamant M, Bendtzen K: Inhibition of production and function of interleukin-6 by 1,25-dihydroxyvitamin D3. *Immunol Lett.* 1991;28(2):115-120.

[31] Cantorna MT, Hayes CE, DeLuca HF: 1,25-Dihydroxyvitamin D3 reversibly blocks the progression of relapsing encephalomyelitis, a model of multiple sclerosis. *Proc Natl Acad. Sci. U S A.* 1996;93(15):7861-7864.

[32] Pedersen LB, Nashold FE, Spach KM, Hayes CE. 1,25-dihydroxyvitamin D3 reverses experimental autoimmune encephalomyelitis by inhibiting chemokine synthesis and monocyte trafficking. *J. Neurosci. Res.* 2007;85(11):2480-2490.

[33] Gorman S, Kuritzky LA, Judge MA, Dixon KM, McGlade JP, Mason RS, Finlay-Jones JJ, Hart PH. Topically applied 1,25-dihydroxyvitamin D3 enhances the suppressive activity of CD4+CD25+ cells in the draining lymph nodes. *J. Immunol.* 2007 Nov 1;179(9):6273-83.

[34] Zhang H, Shih DQ, Zhang X. Mechanisms underlying effects of 1,25-Dihydroxyvitamin D3 on the Th17 cells. *Eur. J. Microbiol. Immunol (Bp).* 2013 Dec;3(4):237-40.

[35] Usategui A, Criado G, Del Rey MJ, Faré R, Pablos JL. Topical vitamin D analogue calcipotriol reduces skin fibrosis in experimental scleroderma. *Arch. Dermatol. Res.* 2014 May 1. [Epub ahead of print]

[36] Cantorna MT, Woodward WD, Hayes CE, DeLuca HF. 1,25-dihydroxyvitamin D3 is a positive regulator for the two anti-encephalitogenic cytokines TGF-beta 1 and IL-4. *J. Immunol.* 1998;160(11):5314-5319.

[37] Deluca HF, Cantorna MT. Vitamin D: its role and uses in immunology. *FASEB J.* 2001 Dec;15(14):2579-85.

[38] Pyzik M, Piccirillo CA: The TGF-beta1/Foxp3 regulatory axis in immune self-tolerance: implications for health and disease. *Inflamm Allergy Drug Targets* 2006;5(3):167-177.

[39] Tran DQ, Ramsey H, Shevach EM. Induction of FOXP3 expression in naive human CD4+FOXP3 T cells by T-cell receptor stimulation is transforming growth factor-beta dependent but does not confer a regulatory phenotype. *Blood* 2007;110(8):2983-2990.

[40] Nashold FE, Nelson CD, Brown LM, Hayes CE. One calcitriol dose transiently increases Helios+ FoxP3+ T cells and ameliorates autoimmune demyelinating disease. *J. Neuroimmunol.* 2013 Oct 15;263(1-2):64-74.

[41] Gabbay MA, Sato MN, Finazzo C, Duarte AJ, Dib SA. Effect of cholecalciferol as adjunctive therapy with insulin on protective immunologic profile and decline of residual β-cell function in new-onset type 1 diabetes mellitus. *Arch. Pediatr. Adolesc. Med.* 2012 Jul 1;166(7):601-7.

[42] Unger WW, Laban S, Kleijwegt FS, van der Slik AR, Roep BO. Induction of Treg by monocyte-derived DC modulated by vitamin D3 or dexamethasone: differential role for PD-L1. *Eur. J. Immunol.* 2009;39(11):3147-3159.

[43] Dong X, Bachman LA, Kumar R, Griffin MD. Generation of antigen-specific, interleukin-10-producing T-cells using dendritic cell stimulation and steroid hormone conditioning. *Transpl. Immunol.* 2003;11(3-4):323-333.

In: Thrombocytopenia
Editor: Mckenzie G. Bell

ISBN: 978-1-63321-713-3

Chapter 4

Thrombocytopenia in Pregnancy

Aisha Hameed **and** ***Sukrutha Veerareddy*** [†]
Queen Elizabeth Hospital, London, UK

Abstract

Platelet counts falls progressively in pregnancy, although usually remains within the lower normal limits. In the third trimester, platelet count can fall to 100x109/l 150x109/l, in the absence of pathological process. Hence, thrombocytopenia is a common finding in pregnancy. Most cases are mild and have no significance for mother or fetus but, in some instances, where thrombocytopenia is part of a complex clinical disorder, there can be profound and even life-threatening consequences for both mother and baby. The commonest cause includes Gestational thrombocytopenia and accounts for 75% of cases of thrombocytopenia in pregnancy and has an incidence upto 8% of all pregnancies. It is a benign condition usually occurs incidentally later in pregnancy and there is no bleeding risk to mother or fetus. Many of the features are similar to mild immune thrombocytopenia (ITP) and it can be difficult to distinguish between the two disorders. There are no specific diagnostic tests for either and both conditions are diagnoses of exclusion.

ITP is usually a chronic condition, often occurring among young women. The incidence is estimated at 0.1-1/1000 pregnancies, accounting for approximately 3% of cases of thrombocytopenia in pregnancy. It is a diagnosis of exclusion, although in approximately two-thirds of cases the diagnosis is already established before pregnancy, allowing the opportunity for pre-pregnancy counselling.

Thrombocytopenia in ITP is predominantly caused by antibodies that are specific to platelet surface glycoproteins - which bind to the platelets in the maternal circulation, resulting in immune-mediated platelet destruction. Recent research suggests there is also suppression of platelet production. The antibodies can cross the placenta and cause fetal thrombocytopenia. The aim of management is to maintain an adequate platelet count that

* Dr Aisha Hameed: Specialist Trainee, Lewisham and Greenwich NHS Trust, Queen Elizabeth Hospital, Stadium Road, SE18 4QH, London. E-mail: aishadr@gmail.com.

† corresponding author: Miss Sukrutha Veerareddy, Consultant Obstetrician and Gynaecologist, Lewisham and Greenwich NHS Trust, Queen Elizabeth Hospital, Stadium Road, SE18 4QH, London. E-mail: Sukrutha. veerareddy@nhs.net.

will minimise the risk of bleeding during pregnancy, delivery and postpartum period. Platelet counts should be closely monitored throughout pregnancy.

The majority of women will not require treatment in the antenatal period, treatment is more often required to increase the count before delivery. Prednisolone is the usual first-line choice but some women may need intravenous immunoglobulin (IVIg) to increase counts rapidly. Rarely, Anti-D immunoglobulin appears be useful for women who are rhesus positive.Both these options are useful when a rapid increase in platelet count is required.

The other rarer causes of thrombocytopenia include Thrombotic thrombocytopenic purpura, Haemolytic Uremic Syndrome, Hereditary Thrombocytopenia, Pseudothrombocytopenia, Viral infection, drugs and lekemia and lymphoma.

Thrombocytopenia in Pregnancy

Introduction

Thrombocytopenia is defined as a platelet count below the 2.5th lower percentile of the normal platelet count distribution. Results of the third US National Health and Nutrition Examination Survey support the traditional value of 150 × 10^9/L as the lower limit of normal. [1] However, platelet counts between 100 and 150 × 10^9/L do not necessarily indicate disease if they have been stable for more than 6 months [2], and the adoption of a cut off value of 100 × 10^9/L may be more appropriate to identify a pathologic condition [3].

Furthermore, it is now appreciated that in many non-Western countries, the lower threshold of the normal platelet count is lower than 150 × 10^9/L [3].

If a low platelet count is seen on an automated complete blood count, spurious thrombocytopenia should be excluded. This phenomenon may occur because of a small clot in the blood sample or platelet clumping caused by the addition of the anticoagulant ethylenediaminetetraacetic acid (EDTA) to the sample.

A repeat count for confirmation and examination of the peripheral blood film can ascertain whether the thrombocytopenia is genuine. If the blood film shows platelet clumps, a repeat complete blood count in a sample anticoagulated with citrate may resolve the problem.

Studies of platelet counts during normal pregnancy differed in their conclusions, with some suggesting no overall effect of pregnancy on platelet count [4-6] and others showing a modest reduction in late pregnancy [6, 7].

One study of platelet counts in 6715 consecutive patients delivering in a single Canadian center showed that thrombocytopenia (platelet count < 150 × 10^9/L) occurred in 7.6% of women, and most (65.1%) had no associated pathology [8]. From a practical point of view, any pregnant woman with a platelet count of less than 100 × 10^9/L in pregnancy should undergo further clinical and laboratory assessment.

All pregnant women with a platelet count less than 150 × 10^9/L after 20 weeks' gestation should have blood pressure and urinalysis checked. In the absence of hypertension or proteinuria, no pathology is found in most women with mild thrombocytopenia at this stage of pregnancy [8].

Obstetrician should determine the pathophysiologic nature of the thrombocytopenia, and risks it poses to both mother and fetus. Treatment depends on gestation, labour and delivery plans.

Causes of Thrombocytopenia in Pregnancy

Isolated Thrombocytopenia	**Part of Systemic disease**
Gestational	Pre eclampcia, HELLP
ITP	Acute Fatty Liver of Pregnancy
Drug Induced	TTP, HUS
Type 2b VWD	Lupus, Antiphospholipid Syndrome
	Viral Infections
	Bone marrow disorders

Pregnancy Specific Common Causes of Thrombocytopenia

First Trimester	**Second Trimester**	**Third Trimester**
ITP	ITP	Gestational
Spurious	PET	PET/HELLP
	Gestational	ITP

Gestational Thrombocytopenia

Gestational Thrombocytopenia is the most common cause of low platelets in pregnancy, responsible for 75% of the cases of thrombocytopenia in pregnancy. There is no indication for induction of labour or pharmacological intervention in Gestational Thrombocytopenia.

Gestational Thrombocytopenia is characterised by asymptomatic thrombocytopenia (Usually above 75 x 10^6 g/l), with no past history of low platelets. It occurs in the third trimester and rarely starts toward the end of second trimester. This does not result in foetal and neonatal thrombocytopenia and resolves spontaneously after delivery. Platelets should be repeated 6 weeks after delivery in community to rule out other causes of low platelets.

ITP (Immune Thrombocytopenia Purpra)

Background

Immune thrombocytopenia (ITP) [8] occurs in one or two of every 1,000 pregnancies [9] and accounts for 5% of cases of pregnancy-associated thrombocytopenia. Factors that induce primary ITP and why its course worsens in some pregnant patients are not well understood. Secondary ITP, develops in association with viral infection (human immunodeficiency virus [HIV], hepatitis C, and Helicobacter pylori) and autoimmune disease.Of all cases of pregnancy-associated ITP, approximately one-third are first diagnosed during pregnancy, whereas two-thirds occur in patients with pre existing disease. Despite its rarity compared to gestational thrombocytopenia, ITP is the most common cause of isolated thrombocytopenia in the first and early second trimesters [3, 6, 9-11].

Pathophysiology of ITP

The pathophysiology of ITP has been classically believed to reflect the accelerated clearance of platelets coated by IgG anti-platelet autoantibodies. These antibodies recognize specific epitopes expressed on platelet glycoproteins such as glycoprotein IIb/IIIa, or less commonly glycoproteins Ib/IX or Ia/IIa [12]. These antibody-coated platelets are then removed following binding to macrophage Fcγ receptors, primarily in the spleen [9, 13-15]. Some antiplatelet antibodies may also directly activate complement [17]. However, recent studies indicate that several other mechanisms also contribute to the pathogenesis of ITP, including diminished platelet production [18, 19] caused at least in part by antibodies that cross react with megakaryocytes [19], and alterations in T cell subsets, in particular loss of regulatory T (Treg) cells [20]. Whether the role of any of these mechanisms is of particular importance in the setting of pregnancy has not been determined.

Signs/Symptoms

The presentation of ITP in pregnancy is much like that in the non-pregnant individual. Patients may be diagnosed following the detection of asymptomatic thrombocytopenia on routine testing, or less commonly with more severe thrombocytopenia accompanied by bruising, bleeding, and petechiae. ITP that predates pregnancy may either worsen or remain quiescent during gestation [21, 22].

Webert et al. reviewed the experience of 92 women with ITP during 119 pregnancies over an 11 year period found that women with previously diagnosed ITP were less likely to require therapy for ITP than those with newly diagnosed ITP [23].

Diagnosis

As in the non-pregnant state, the diagnosis of ITP is a clinical diagnosis of exclusion. [16].The likelihood that a patient suffers from ITP rather than incidental thrombocytopenia of pregnancy increases as the platelet count decreases; however, no specific platelet count below which incidental thrombocytopenia may be excluded has been defined.[16] Many patients with apparent incidental thrombocytopenia have elevated levels of platelet-associated IgG, platelet antibody tests do not differentiate these syndromes [24]. In a large study utilizing the monoclonal antibody-specific immobilization of platelet-antigens (MAPA) assay, less than 7% of thrombocytopenic pregnant women were found to have autoantibodies, and there was no significant difference in the prevalence of autoantibodies between thrombocytopenic and non-thrombocytopenic pregnant women [24-27]. Thus, the most useful means of differentiating these syndromes is, by definition, the antenatal history [28, 29].

A history of prior thrombocytopenia, underlying autoimmune disease or severe thrombocytopenia (< 50,000/μl) makes the diagnosis of ITP more likely. In the absence of a platelet count prior to pregnancy, significant thrombocytopenia in the first trimester, with a declining platelet count as gestation progresses, is most consistent with ITP. In contrast, mild thrombocytopenia developing in the second or third trimester and not associated with hypertension or proteinuria most likely represents incidental thrombocytopenia [11].

Other relevant questions that should be assessed when evaluating a pregnant patient with thrombocytopenia include whether prior deliveries were complicated by excessive bleeding, and whether the infant had thrombocytopenia or bleeding complications. The physical examination should focus on excluding secondary causes of thrombocytopenia.

For example, elevated blood pressure and/or the onset of peripheral edema or weight gain may suggest thrombocytopenia complicating a pregnancy-associated hypertensive disorder [30]. In addition, symptoms potentially consistent with the early development of the HELLP syndrome, such as right upper quadrant pain, increasing malaise or severe headache should be specifically sought [31, 32].

Finally, all thrombocytopenic pregnant patients should be carefully evaluated for the presence of risk factors for HIV and HCV infection [33].

Laboratory investigation of the pregnant patient with suspected ITP should include a complete blood count and platelet count.[16] Examination of the peripheral blood film is essential to exclude not only pseudothrombocytopenia, but other thrombocytopenic disorders such as TTP or preeclampsia, in which the peripheral blood film may reveal increased numbers of fragmented red cells [30]. Other studies that should be considered include liver enzyme tests, urinalysis, and HIV and HCV testing. Bone marrow examination is not recommended unless other hematologic abnormalities (other than mild pregnancy-associated anemia) or unusual findings on physical examination are identified. As in non-pregnant individuals, a lack of response to standard ITP therapy in a pregnant patient with thrombocytopenia should prompt consideration of a bone marrow examination.[16]

Management

The clinical management of pregnancy-associated ITP should be multidisciplinary, requiring close collaboration between the obstetrician, haematologist, specialist midwife and anaesthetist (toward delivery). Pregnant women with ITP require careful monitoring, and should be seen monthly in the first and second trimester, every 2 weeks after 28 weeks, and weekly after 36 weeks.[16] Visits should involve routine obstetrical care with emphasis on blood pressure, weight, urine dipstick analysis for protein, and serial platelet counts i.e signs and symptoms of pre eclampcia should be clearly sought. Decisions concerning the need for therapy are determined primarily by the patient's symptoms, particularly whether active bleeding is present, though the absolute platelet count should be considered as term approaches with the potential need for epidural anaesthesia.[16] The American Society of Haematology (ASH) and British Committee for Standards of Haematology (BCSH) guidelines consider treatment to be appropriate for severe thrombocytopenia and/or thrombocytopenia associated with bleeding.

However, though there is no evidence to support the opinion that platelet counts should be kept higher in the asymptomatic pregnant woman than in other thrombocytopenic patients [34]. More aggressive treatment is recommended later in pregnancy to prepare the patient for labor and delivery, which often is accompanied by the use of epidural anaesthesia.[16]

Treatment has been recommended for women with a platelet count below 10,000/μl at any time during pregnancy, or below 30,000/μl in the second or third trimester or when associated with bleeding [35-37]. There is lack of consensus in regard to treatment of patients with a platelet count of <30,000/μl but no bleeding in the first trimester, reflecting the desire to avoid exposure of such patients to corticosteroids during pregnancy [37, 38]. Though treatment of the pregnant woman with ITP generally does not differ significantly from that of non-pregnant individuals, there are some unique considerations [39-42]. Due to their efficacy and low cost, many consider corticosteroids to be first line treatment for ITP in pregnancy [36]. The mechanisms of action of corticosteroids are due, at least in part, to the inhibition of phagocytosis of opsonized platelets, as well as impairment of autoantibody production. The typical therapeutic dose of prednisone is 1 mg/kg/day (based on the pre-pregnancy weight), which, after achieving a response, is gradually titrated to the lowest effective dose.

However, the many adverse effects of corticosteroids are amplified during pregnancy, and pregnancy-specific complications such as gestational diabetes, weight gain, acceleration of bone loss, hypertension and premature labor must be recognized [7, 38]. Furthermore, some studies have associated the use of corticosteroids in the first trimester with congenital anomalies, such as orofacial clefts [44, 45]. Due to above serious suspected complications in the women in whom therapy is indicated but not urgent, initiation of corticosteroid therapy at a low dose, perhaps 20-30 mg/day of prednisone, should be considered. Alternatively, others have suggested that IVIg should be the first line therapy for pregnancy-associated ITP, especially when a long duration of therapy may not be required [11]. So therapy should be individualized according to the need of that particular patient.

Treatment with high dose (i.e. 2 gm/kg over 2-5 days) IVIg is an effective means of raising the platelet count rapidly.[16] Compared to corticosteroids, IVIg is less likely to induce toxicities such as hypertension [23, 24]. ASH guidelines consider IVIg to be an appropriate first line agent for severe thrombocytopenia, or thrombocytopenic bleeding in the third trimester. Woman's informed consent should be sought before administration of IVIG. However, responses to IVIg tend to be transient, and multiple courses of therapy may be required at significant cost and patient inconvenience. A subset of patients who fail to respond satisfactorily to corticosteroids or IVIg alone may respond to high doses of these agents when administered in combination (methylprednisolone 1gm, IVIg 1-2gm/kg) [2, 10].

Splenectomy may be considered albeit rarely as another option for patients who fail to adequately respond to corticosteroids or IVIg. Remission of ITP is initially achieved in approximately 75% of pregnant women who undergo splenectomy. Splenectomy should be ideally performed in the second trimester, as surgery earlier in pregnancy may induce miscarriage, and later in pregnancy splenectomy may be technically difficult due to obstruction of the surgical field by the gravid uterus [2-4]. Laparoscopic splenectomy has been safely performed in pregnant women.[16]

In patients who develop severe ITP refractory to steroids and IVIG, and who are beyond the second trimester, which could be optimum time for splenectomy, intravenous anti-D has been used successfully.In one report, 6 of 8 women who received anti-D in their second and third trimester had partial responses, with no major maternal or fetal complications, and no evidence of hydrops.[48].Safety of Anti D in pregnancy is still questionable[16]

Other agents used to treat ITP in the non-pregnant population, namely cytotoxic and immunosuppressive agents, are potential teratogens. For this reason, danazol, cyclophosphamide and vinca alkaloids should be avoided in pregnancy.[16] Azathioprine has been used safely in pregnant patients with renal transplants. However, neonatal hematologic and immune impairment have been reported in some exposed infants and azathioprine remains a category D agent. Rituximab has been used in several pregnant patients with lymphoma. No major fetal malformations have been associated with its use, though infants born to mothers treated with this agent may experience abnormal B-lymphocyte development in their first year of life. In a few case reports, immunologic recovery was observed at 6 months of life with no infection-related complications. Due to the lack of sufficient evidence of safety, Kimbey et al. recommend that Rituximab be avoided in the treatment of pregnancy-associated ITP. Thus, in general, the use of cytotoxic and immunosuppressive agents should be limited to severe cases refractory to other treatments. These agents should be used in the second and third trimesters only and each case should be considered individually.[16]

There is very little experience with either of the thrombopoietic agents in pregnancy, and both are contraindicated for this indication. A pregnancy registry has been developed for patients who become pregnant while taking either Eltrombopag or Romiplostim. Likewise it is not known whether either of these agents are excreted in human milk, and thus their safety in nursing mothers has not been established.

Management of Delivery

Cesaerean section is only indicated for obstetrics reasons. In terms of maternal management, the primary consideration is achieving a platelet count sufficient to minimize maternal hemorrhage during vaginal delivery and cesarean section. Epidural anesthesia is also commonly used during labour, and adequate hemostasis is required to minimize the risk of any resulting neurologic complications that might arise. The American Society of Hematology guidelines suggest that a maternal platelet count of 50,000/µl is sufficient for vaginal delivery as well as cesarean section. But British guidelines recommend that a platelet count of 80,000/µl be attained for cesarean delivery as well as for epidural anesthesia, based on a retrospective review in which epidural anesthesia was successfully delivered with no neurologic complications in 30 thrombocytopenic women with platelet counts between 69,000-98,000/µl. It will be interesting to look at American data of the women who received Spinal or Epidural Anaesthesia during labour or delivery with platelet between 50,000/µl and 80,000/µl If there are no complications, which most likely is the case, British Society of Haematology can reconsider their criteria. Thus, though no prospective, randomized data is available to address this issue definitively, most experts consider a platelet count in the range of 80,000/µl adequate for epidural anesthesia and either vaginal delivery or cesarean section in the parturient. Since this may be significantly higher than the therapeutic platelet count range targeted earlier in pregnancy, additional therapy may be required in some pregnant patients as term approaches.[16]

Considerations should be given to the fetal platelet count and the risk of intracranial hemorrhage during delivery.[16] Maternal IgG is actively transported to the fetal circulation subsequent to its binding to Fcγ receptors on the syncytiotrophoblast cells of the placenta. These maternal platelet-reactive antibodies may cross-react with antigens on fetal platelets, leading to the development of fetal thrombocytopenia, which is associated with an increased risk for hemorrhage during delivery.[16] In a large metaanalysis that reviewed series containing 10 or more patients in whom fetal platelet counts were determined, 288 live-born infants were identified. Platelet counts below 50,000/µl were observed in 10.1% of these infants, while platelet counts below 20,000/µl occurred in 4.2%.[50]

The risk of fetal intracranial hemorrhage in the fetus of patients with ITP is very low. Risk of intracranial hemorrhage, which in theory, has been expected to be increased by head trauma occurring during passage of the fetus through the birth canal during vaginal delivery. In a large observational study, the incidence of intracranial hemorrhage was below 1% [38]. In this report, the course of 284 mothers with ITP and their 286 newborn infants was described [38]. Neonatal thrombocytopenia (platelet count <100,000/µl) was diagnosed in 22.6% of the offspring, though only 6.3% experienced bleeding events, and there were no episodes of intracranial hemorrhage. There was no correlation between platelet counts or the ITP status of the mothers and the development of neonatal thrombocytopenia, an observation that has been reported in almost all studies that have examined this issue. Indeed, there is no consistent or reproducible correlation between the fetal platelet count at delivery and a number of maternal characteristics including the severity of maternal thrombocytopenia [10, 11], or the level of circulating maternal antiplatelet IgG [29].

The most reliable predictor of neonatal thrombocytopenia is a history of thrombocytopenia at delivery in a prior sibling.[49]

Due to the inability to predict neonatal thrombocytopenia based on maternal clinical characteristics, invasive procedures such as fetal scalp sampling during labor, or percutaneous umbilical blood sampling (PUBS) have been developed.[16] Fetal scalp vein sampling (FBS) is technically difficult; platelet counts obtained through this procedure have not been shown to correlate with the platelet count at delivery and may falsely predict thrombocytopenia, possibly due to clotting of blood during sampling.[16] In contrast, PUBS is often able to yield accurate platelet counts, but is associated with complication rates of up to 2%, approximately half of which may necessitate emergent delivery and ultimately result in pregnancy loss. Thus, the risks of fetal platelet count determination are at the least equal to, and likely exceed that of fetal intracranial hemorrhage, negating its clinical utility [34].

While it was previously believed that cesarean section reduced the risk of fetal intracranial hemorrhage during delivery of offspring of patients with ITP, studies over the last two decades have demonstrated that this does not appear to be the case [11]. In one study, 31 pregnancies in 25 women with ITP over a 10 year period were reviewed. Fourteen infants were born vaginally, and 18 by cesarean, with no complications in any, despite platelet counts below 100,000/µl in 5 infants, and below 50,000/µl in 2 of them. These authors also reviewed literature reports of 474 infants born to mothers with ITP, finding that platelet counts below 50,000/µl occurred in 15%, and intracranial hemorrhage in 3%. However, no association of intracranial hemorrhage with the mode of delivery was observed.

In another retrospective review of 601 infants of mothers with ITP, severe neonatal thrombocytopenia was reported in 72 (12%), with relatively equal numbers of these babies being delivered by vaginal delivery (n=307) or cesarean section (n=247). Six infants developed intracranial hemorrhage, two of which were delivered by cesarean section. Four of these six infants had severe neonatal thrombocytopenia [29].

Thus, given the fact that neonatal intracranial hemorrhage is an extremely rare complication of maternal ITP, and that cesarean deliveries may be associated with significant maternal morbidity, it is generally recommended that cesarean section be performed only for maternal indications.

Following delivery, serial platelet counts should be obtained in all newborns at birth and during the first week postpartum, because the onset of thrombocytopenia due to maternal anti-platelet IgG may be delayed. In a study of 61 infants born to ITP mothers, 66% of neonates experienced a further fall in their platelet counts after birth, with 54% reaching their nadir by day 2. The platelet count stabilized or began to rise by day 7 in all infants.[45]

ASH guidelines suggest that infants with a platelet count below 20,000/µl, or those with hemorrhage, receive treatment. IVIg at a dose of 1gm/kg is effective in inducing a prompt rise in the platelet count; the concurrent use of corticosteroids is controversial due to a possible predisposition to neonatal sepsis.

Imaging of the brain with ultrasonography, computed tomography or magnetic resonance should be performed in all newborns with platelet counts of less than 50,000/µl to exclude the possibility of occult intracranial hemorrhage that may require prompt intervention.

Postpartum Management

Women with ITP should not be discouraged from breast feeding, as there has been no firm association established between breast feeding and neonatal thrombocytopenia [43].

Postpartum thromboprophylaxis should be offered according to VTE scoring, Low Molecular Weight Heparin (LMWH) can be given in women with platelets above $50x10^9/L$, if platelets are below this level graduated compression stockings should be used. Non steroidal anti-inflammatory drugs should be strictly avoided.

Thrombocytopenia in Systemic Disease

Thrombotic Thrombocytopenia Purpura TTP

TTP is a rare disorder with platelet activation that leads to platelet thrombi in microcirculation. Clinical features are thrombocytopenia, impaired renal functions, microangiopathic hemolysis, neurological features and fever. It has different pathophysiology from HUS, but they have quite a few of common/overlapping features. The incidence of TTP/HUS among all pregnancies has been estimated to be 1 in 25 000 [44], significantly more frequent than in the general population [45] The time of onset of TTP/HUS in pregnancy is variable, but only a minority of cases are seen during the first trimester.

TTP is associated with a deficiency of ADAMTS13 (a disintegrin and metalloproteinase with a thrombospondin type 1 motif, member 13), which is rarely congenital and inherited (Upshaw-Schulman syndrome) and may manifest for the first time during pregnancy.

Early diagnosis of TTP/HUS is essential to institute treatment promptly because most fatal events occur within 24 hours from presentation in untreated subjects [46] Any patient with thrombocytopenia and microangiopathic hemolytic anemia in the absence of any obvious precipitating condition should be classified as TTP/HUS.

Laboratory findings reveal evidence of microangiopathic hemolytic anemia, a negative (with rare exceptions) direct antiglobulin test, and normal coagulation tests (prothrombin time, activated partial thromboplastin time, fibrinogen and D-dimers).

Renal impairment may be revealed by raised creatinine levels, with urinalysis often revealing only mild proteinuria, microscopic hematuria, and few casts.

Maternal and Fetal Complications

Untreated TTP can be fatal for mother and fetus. Plasma exchange with Fresh Frozen Plasma improves the outcome of both. Unlike HELLP and AFLP delivery does not need to be expedited as it does not change the outlook unless it is accompanied by pre eclampcia.

Plasma exchange is initially performed daily until the platelet count is $> 150 \times 10^9/L$ for at least 3 days and serum LDH concentrations have returned to normal, or nearly normal, levels. We gradually taper off plasma exchange over a 2-week period.

British guidelines suggest starting aspirin 75 mg/d and low molecular weight heparin at prophylactic doses (e.g. dalteparin 5000 IU/d subcutaneously) once the platelet count is $> 50 \times 10^9/L$; these recommendations, however, are not routinely followed in other countries. If TTP develops in the first trimester, regular plasma exchange may allow continuation of pregnancy with delivery of a live infant.

The frequency of the exchanges is guided by blood counts and serum lactate dehydrogenase (LDH) concentrations. Delivery is recommended for women who do not respond to plasma exchange.

Pre Eclampcia and HELLP Syndrome

Background

Pre-eclampcia is a pregnancy specific disorder, it is mutisystemic complex, unpredictable and has variable manifestation. Diffuse endothelial damage causes widespread damage to liver, hepatic, cardiovascular, nervous system and coagulation system. Classical signs are hypertension, proteinurea and biochemical abnormalities.

Biochemical abnormalities include raised liver transaminases, raised creatinine and low platelets. HELLP is a variant or complication of pre eclampcia.

Preeclampsia, defined by criteria established by NICE (National Institute of Clinical Excellence) affects up to 6% of all first pregnancies and is the most common cause of pregnancy-associated mortality worldwide. Criteria for the diagnosis of preeclampsia include the following: (i) blood pressure of 140 mm Hg systolic or 90 mm Hg diastolic or higher that occurs after 20 weeks of gestation in a woman with previously normal blood pressure; and (ii) proteinuria, defined as urinary excretion of 0.3 grams of protein or higher in a 24-hour specimen, that usually correlates with a 1+ or greater reading on dipstick.

Multiple organ systems are affected in preeclampsia, reflecting systemic endothelial dysfunction, although the kidneys are affected most severely. Predisposing factors include primiparity, age < 20 years or > 35 years, raised body mass index, chronic hypertension, and a gestational or pre pregnancy Diabetes.

Thrombocytopenia occurs in up to 50% of women with preeclampsia, and its severity generally parallels that of the underlying preeclampsia. Importantly, thrombocytopenia may occasionally precede other manifestations of preeclampsia, and thus preeclampsia must be considered in the differential diagnosis of isolated thrombocytopenia developing in the late second or third trimester.

Pathophysiology

It is interesting to note that the clinical manifestations of preeclampsia usually do not appear until the late second or third trimester, the pathologic processes underlying this syndrome reflect inadequate placentation early in pregnancy. In preeclampsia, both the depth of trophoblast invasion and the extent of remodeling of the spiral arteries are reduced; this may reflect deficiencies in trophoblast function, including failure of trophoblast cells to alter their pattern of integrin expression toward an endothelial phenotype and deficient protease activity, among others. Insufficient placentation results in progressive ischemia of the fetoplacental unit as pregnancy advances, and fetal growth and oxygen requirements increase. It has been postulated that placental hypoperfusion which in turn releases various factors that trigger endothelial activation/dysfunction.

A recent study has identified that low levels of PIGF (Placental growth Factor) in maternal blood can accurately predict the chances of developing severe PET in the women with accuracy of 90%. A large trial is underway.

Sign/Symptoms

Criteria for the HELLP syndrome vary somewhat among studies, but generally include microangiopathic hemolytic anemia, a lactate dehydrogenase (LDH) > 600 U/mL, increased aspartate aminotransferase (≥ 40-70 U/mL, depending on the series), and thrombocytopenia (platelet count < 100,000/μL. Unlike preeclampsia, HELLP is more common in multiparous women. Approximately 70% of cases of HELLP occur prior to term, with the remainder usually occurring within 48 hours after delivery. Up to 75% of patients with HELLP have proteinuria, but only 50% to 60% have hypertension. Patients with HELLP frequently present with malaise, accompanied by severe right upper quadrant pain thought to result from obstruction of blood flow in the hepatic sinusoids; liver pathology confirms hepatocyte necrosis with fibrin deposition in periportal sinusoids. A wide differential diagnosis must be considered in patients presenting with HELLP, including intraabdominal processes such as nephrolithiasis, cholecystitis, and appendicitis, among others. A recent study identified mutations in genes regulating the activity of the alternative complement system (factor H, factor I, and membrane cofactor protein) in 4 of 11 patients with HELLP, suggesting that, as in atypical hemolytic uremic syndrome (HUS), excessive complement activation may be involved in the pathogenesis of HELLP in some patients.

Management

The general approach to therapy for these disorders in women beyond 34 weeks is stabilization, followed by expeditious delivery of the fetus. At earlier points in pregnancy, delivery may be undertaken following administration of betamethasone to enhance fetal lung maturity, although some advocate expectant therapy in selected patients as a means to improve fetal outcome. Both disorders generally begin to remit within several days after delivery, although in some individuals, in particular those with HELLP, prolonged thrombocytopenia and elevations of LDH lasting for as long as several weeks may occur postpartum. HELLP and preeclampsia may also uncommonly present postpartum.

A patient with preeclampsia or HELLP is at increased risk for development of recurrent disease and poor pregnancy outcome in subsequent pregnancies, particularly if the initial disorder occurred with an early onset. According to NICE guidelines risk of recurrence in 25% if a women develops severe PET, HELLP or early onset IUGR needing delivery before 34 weeks in subsequent pregnancy and it increases upto 55% if PET necessitate delivery before 28 weeks. Several large clinical trials have utilized agents such as aspirin or antioxidants such as vitamins C and E, in attempts to prevent preeclampsia, particularly in high-risk individuals. A meta-analysis suggests that aspirin has modest efficacy in prevention of preeclampsia, although no difference in the incidence of fetal death was demonstrated. Patients with preeclampsia are at increased risk for cardiovascular disease in long-term follow-up. After delivery of the baby, platelets resume to normal slowly.

References

[1] Cheng, C. K., Chan, J., Cembrowski, G. S., and van Assendelft, O. W. (2004) Complete blood count reference interval diagrams derived from NHANES III: stratification by age, sex, and race. *Lab. Hematol.* 10(1):42-53.

[2] Stasi, R., Amadori, S., Osborn, J., Newland, A. C., and Provan, D. (2006) Long-term outcome of otherwise healthy individuals with incidentally discovered borderline thrombocytopenia. *PLoS Med.* 3(3):e24.

[3] Rodeghiero, F., Stasi, R., Gernsheimer, T., et al. (2009) Standardization of terminology, definitions and outcome criteria in immune thrombocytopenic purpura of adults and children: report from an international working group. *Blood* 113(11):2386-2393.

[4] British Committee for Standards in Haematology: General Haematology Task Force guidelines for the investigation and management of idiopathic thrombocytopenic purpura in adults, children and in pregnancy. *Br. J. Haematol.*

[5] Clark, A. L., Gall, S. A.: Clinical uses of intravenous immunoglobulin in pregnancy. *Am. J. Obstet. Gynecol.* 176:241-

[6] Godeau, B., Chevret, S., Varet, B., et al.: for the French ITP Study Group: Intravenous immunoglobulin or high dose methylprednisolone, with or without oral prednisolone, for adults with untreated severe autoimmune thrombocytopenic purpura: A randomized multicentre trial. *Lancet.* 359:23-29 2002.

[7] Laffan, M., Brown, S. A., Collins, P. W., et al.: The diagnosis of von Willebrand disease: A guideline from the UK Haemophilia Centre Doctors Organisation. *Haemophilia.* 10:199-217 2004.

[8] Cines, D. B., Bussel, J. B., Liebman, H. A., et al. The ITP syndrome: pathogenic and clinical diversity. *Blood.* 2009.

[9] Provan, D., Newland, A. Idiopathic thrombocytopenic purpura in adults. *J. Pediatr. Hematol. Oncol.* 2003;25(Suppl. 1):S34.

[10] McCrae, K. R., Samuels, P., Schreiber, A. D. Pregnancy-associated thrombocytopenia: pathogenesis and management. *Blood.* 1992;80(11):2697.

[11] Gill, K. K., Kelton, J. G. Management of idiopathic thrombocytopenic purpura in pregnancy. *Semin. Hematol.* 2000;37(3):275.

[12] McMillan, R. Immune-mediated thrombocytopenias: focus on chronic immune thrombocytopenic purpura. *Semin. Hematol.* 2007;44(4 Suppl. 5):S1.

[13] Baldini, M. Idiopathic thrombocytopenic purpura. *N. Engl. J. Med.* 1966;274(24):1360.

[14] Cines, D. B., Blanchette, V. S. Immune thrombocytopenic purpura. *N. Engl. J. Med.* 2002; 346(13):995.

[15] Harrington, W. J., Minnich, V., Hollingsworth, J. W., et al. Demonstration of a thrombocytopenic factor in the blood of patients with thrombocytopenic purpura. *J. Lab. Clin. Med.* 1951;38(1):1.

[16] Stavrou E,McCrae KR Immune thrombocytopenia in pregnancy. Hematol Oncol Clin North Am **23**:1299–1316.

[17] Cines, D. B., Schreiber, A. D. Immune thrombocytopenia. Use of a Coombs antiglobulin test to detect IgG and C3 on platelets. *N. Engl. J. Med.* 1979;300(3):106.

[18] Chang, M., Nakagawa, P. A., Williams, S. A., et al. Immune thrombocytopenic purpura (ITP) plasma and purified ITP monoclonal autoantibodies inhibit megakaryocytopoiesis in vitro. *Blood.* 2003;102(3):887.

[19] McMillan, R., Wang, L., Tomer, A., et al. Suppression of in vitro megakaryocyte production by antiplatelet autoantibodies from adult patients with chronic ITP. *Blood.* 2004;103(4):1364.

[20] McMillan, R. The pathogenesis of chronic immune thrombocytopenic purpura. *Semin. Hematol.* 2007;44(4 Suppl. 5):S3.

[21] Devendra, K., Koh, L. P. Pregnancy in women with idiopathic thrombocytopaenic purpura. *Ann. Acad. Med. Singapore*. 2002;31(3):276.

[22] Won, Y. W., Moon, W., Yun, Y. S., et al. Clinical aspects of pregnancy and delivery in patients with chronic idiopathic thrombocytopenic purpura (ITP) *Korean J. Intern. Med.* 2005;20(2):129.

[23] Webert, K. E., Mittal, R., Sigouin, C., et al. A retrospective 11-year analysis of obstetric patients with idiopathic thrombocytopenic purpura. *Blood*. 2003;102(13):4306.

[24] Boehlen, F., Hohlfeld, P., Extermann, P., et al. Maternal antiplatelet antibodies in predicting risk of neonatal thrombocytopenia. *Obstet. Gynecol.* 1999;93(2):169.

[25] Shehata, N., Burrows, R., Kelton, J. G. Gestational thrombocytopenia. *Clin. Obstet. Gynecol.* 1999;42(2):327.

[26] Sainio, S., Kekomaki, R., Riikonen, S., et al. Maternal thrombocytopenia at term: a population-based study. *Acta Obstet. Gynecol. Scand*. 2000;79(9):744.

[27] Samuels, P., Main, E. K., Tomaski, A., et al. Abnormalities in platelet antiglobulin tests in preeclamptic mothers and their neonates. *Am. J. Obstet. Gynecol.* 1987;157(1):109.

[28] Burrows, R. F., Kelton, J. G. Incidentally detected thrombocytopenia in healthy mothers and their infants. *N. Engl. J. Med.* 1988;319(3):142.

[29] Samuels, P., Bussel, J. B., Braitman, L. E., et al. Estimation of the risk of thrombocytopenia in the offspring of pregnant women with presumed immune thrombocytopenic purpura. *N. Engl. J. Med.* 1990;323(4):229.

[30] Pridjian, G., Puschett, J. B. Preeclampsia. Part 1: clinical and pathophysiologic considerations. *Obstet. Gynecol. Surv*. 2002;57(9):598.

[31] O'Brien, J. M., Barton, J. R. Controversies with the diagnosis and management of HELLP syndrome. *Clin. Obstet. Gynecol*. 2005;48(2):460.

[32] Barton, J. R., Sibai, B. M. Diagnosis and management of hemolysis, elevated liver enzymes, and low platelets syndrome. *Clin. Perinatol*. 2004;31(4):807.

[33] Nardi, M., Karpatkin, S. Antiidiotype antibody against platelet anti-GPIIIa contributes to the regulation of thrombocytopenia in HIV-1-ITP patients. *J. Exp. Med.* 2000; 191 (12):2093.

[34] Ajzenberg, N., Dreyfus, M., Kaplan, C., et al. Pregnancy-associated thrombocytopenia revisited: assessment and follow-up of 50 cases. *Blood*. 1998;92(12):4573.

[35] Letsky, E. A., Greaves, M. Guidelines on the investigation and management of thrombocytopenia in pregnancy and neonatal alloimmune thrombocytopenia. Maternal and Neonatal Haemostasis Working Party of the Haemostasis and Thrombosis Task Force of the British Society for Haematology. *Br. J. Haematol.* 1996;95(1):21.

[36] George, J. N., Woolf, S. H., Raskob, G. E., et al. Idiopathic thrombocytopenic purpura: a practice guideline developed by explicit methods for the American Society of Hematology. *Blood*. 1996;88(1):3.

[37] Guidelines for the investigation and management of idiopathic thrombocytopenic purpura in adults, children and in pregnancy. *British Journal of Haematology*. 2003; 120(4):574.

[38] Fujimura, K., Harada, Y., Fujimoto, T., et al. Nationwide study of idiopathic thrombocytopenic purpura in pregnant women and the clinical influence on neonates. *Int. J. Hematol.* 2002;75(4):426.

[39] Kelton, J. G. Management of the pregnant patient with idiopathic thrombocytopenic purpura. *Ann. Intern. Med.* 1983;99(6):796.

[40] Carloss, H. W., McMillan, R., Crosby, W. H. Management of pregnancy in women with immune thrombocytopenic purpura. *JAMA*. 1980;244(24):2756.

[41] Moise, K. J., Jr Autoimmune thrombocytopenic purpura in pregnancy. *Clin. Obstet. Gynecol.* 1991;34(1):51.

[42] Kessler, I., Lancet, M., Borenstein, R., et al. The obstetrical management of patients with immunologic thrombocytopenic purpura. *Int. J. Gynaecol. Obstet.* 1982;20(1):23.

[43] Christiaens, G. C., Nieuwenhuis, H. K., von dem Borne, A. E., et al. Idiopathic thrombocytopenic purpura in pregnancy: a randomized trial on the effect of antenatal low dose corticosteroids on neonatal platelet count. *Br. J. Obstet. Gynaecol.* 1990;97 (10):893.

[44] Dashe, J. S., Ramin, S. M., Cunningham, F. G. The long-term consequences of thrombotic microangiopathy (thrombotic thrombocytopenic purpura and hemolytic uremic syndrome) in pregnancy. *Obstet. Gynecol.* 1998;91(5):662-668.

[45] Terrell, D. R., Beebe, L. A., Vesely, S. K., Neas, B. R., Segal, J. B., George, J. N. The incidence of immune thrombocytopenic purpura in children and adults: a critical review of published reports. *Am. J. Hematol.* 2010;85(3):174-180.

[46] Scully, M., Yarranton, H., Liesner, R., et al. Regional UK TTP registry: correlation with laboratory ADAMTS 13 analysis and clinical features. *Br. J. Haematol.* 2008; 142 (5):819-826.

[47] George, J. N. How I treat patients with thrombotic thrombocytopenic purpura: 2010. *Blood* 2010;116(20):4060-4069.

[48] Cines DB, Bussel JB. How I treat idiopathic thrombocytopenic purpura (ITP) Blood. 2005;106(7):2244.

[49] CHRISTIAENS GCML, NIEUWENHUIS HK, BUSSEL JB. Comparison of Platelet Counts in First and Second Newborns of Mothers With Immune Thrombocytopenic Purpura. Obstetrics & Gynecology. 1997;90(4 Part 1):546

[50] Burrows RF, Kelton JG. Pregnancy in patients with idiopathic thrombocytopenic purpura: assessing the risks for the infant at delivery. Obstet Gynecol Surv. 1993;48(12):781

In: Thrombocytopenia
Editor: Mckenzie G. Bell

ISBN: 978-1-63321-713-3

Chapter 5

Differential Diagnosis of Thrombocytopenia

Libor Červinek and Michael Doubek*
Department of Internal Medicine – Hematology and Oncology,
University Hospital and Masaryk University, Brno, Czech Republic

Abstract

Decreased platelet counts can be due to a number of disease processes causing decreased platelet production, increased platelet destruction, or can be medication-induced. We have to differentiate inherited thrombocytopenias, primary immune thrombocytopenias (ITP), secondary immune thrombocytopenias, myelodysplastic syndromes with thrombocytopenia, bone marrow failure syndromes and non-immune thrombocytopenias. ITP is the most common cause of isolated thrombocytopenia.

There are three diagnostic cornerstones for diagnosing ITP – patient history, physical examination, and peripheral blood smear confirming thrombocytopenia to exclude pseudothrombocytopenia. Other tests recommended to establish ITP diagnosis are direct antiglobulin test and tests for *Helicobacter pylori*, HIV and hepatitis C.

Introduction

Decreased platelet counts (less than 100 x 10^9/L) can be due to a number of disease processes causing decreased platelet production, increased platelet destruction, or can be medication-induced. We have to differentiate inherited thrombocytopenias, primary immune thrombocytopenias (ITP), secondary immune thrombocytopenias, myelodysplastic syndromes with thrombocytopenia, bone marrow failure syndromes and non-immune thrombocytopenias. Therefore, complex differential diagnosis of thrombocytonpenia should be carried out.

* Corresponding author: Michael Doubek, MD, PhD, University Hospital, Jihlavská 20, 62500 Brno, Czech Republic.

Symptoms

Often, low platelet levels do not lead to clinical problems; rather, they are picked up on a routine complete blood count. Occasionally, bleeding is the thrombocytopenia symptom. There may be bruising, particularly purpura, petechia in the forearms and legs, epistaxis or bleeding gums. A person with thrombocytopenia may also complain of malaise, fatigue, and general weakness (with or without accompanying blood loss).

Inspection typically reveals evidence of bleeding (petechiae or ecchymoses), along with slow, continuous bleeding from any injuries or wounds.

The bleeding usually occurs when the platelet count is below 30×10^9/L [2].

Diagnostic Procedures

Medical history and physical examination are key procedures to uncover the cause of thrombocytopenia. The haematologist has to study the patient's full medical history prior to this bleeding manifestation very carefully. The patient's history is helpful in the course of invasive surgical procedures, pregnancy, delivery and tooth brushing. The Patient's medical history is also required to exclude common causes of thrombocytopenia like drug associated thrombocytopenia - eg. heparin, quinidine, antibiotics, gold salts, carbamazepine, valproic acid. Other common causes of thrombocytopenia are pregnancy or gestation thrombocytopenia, infection, vaccination and alcoholism [2-4]. Confirmation of thrombocytopenia is the first step in diagnosis. We have to perform complete blood count analysis and evaluate the platelets using microscopy. There should be changes in platelet appearance in some thrombocytopenias. Large platelets are common in patients with immune thrombocytopenia. Giant platelets can be seen in patient with Ph negative myeloproliferative diseases and in patients with inherited thrombocytopenias (Bernard Soulier syndrome, May-Hegglin anomaly). Every new patient with low platelet count without manifest bleeding is suspected of having pseudothrombocytopenia. Microscopic evaluation excludes pseudothrombocytopenia due to EDTA anticoagulants or platelet satellitism. Laboratory tests might also include: biochemistry (liver enzymes, renal function, vitamin B12 levels, folic acid levels) and peripheral blood smear. If the cause of the low platelet count remains unclear, a bone marrow analysis is usually recommended to differentiate whether the low platelet count is due to decreased production or peripheral destruction [3-5]. Analyzing platelet antigens using flow-cytometry can help in differential diagnosis of inherited thrombocytopenias.

Selected Causes of Thrombocytopenia

Inherited Thrombocytopenias

Some disorders of platelet number and function are inherited eg. X-linked Wiskott-Aldrich syndrome which is predominantly present in male patients [5-7]. Other forms of inherited thrombocytopenias are listed in Table 1.

These thrombocytopenias are divided according to platelet size.

Table 1. List of inherited thrombocytopenias

Thrombocytopenia with small platelet size	
Wiscott-Aldrich syndrome (X-linked)	X-linked, severe imunodeficiency
X-linked thrombocytopenia	X-linked, no or mild Immunodeficiency
Thrombocytopenia with normal platelet size	
Congenital amegakaryocytic thrombocytopenia	AR, reduced megakaryocytes in bone marrow, evolution to bone marrow failure
Amegakaryocytic thrombocytopenia with radioulnar synostosis	AD, reduced megakaryocytes, occasional evolution to aplastic anemia
Thrombocytopenia with absent radii	AR, reduced megakaryocytes in bone marrow
Familial platelet disorder and predisposition to acute myeloid leukemia	AD, increased risk to acute myelogenous leukemia
ANKRD36-related thrombocytopenia	AD
Thrombocytopenia and large platelet size	
MYH9-related disease (eg. May-Hegglin anomaly)	AD, leukocyte inclusions, cataracts, nefrropathy, deafnes
Platelet-type von Willebrandt disease	AD
Bernard-Soulier syndrome	AR or AD
Gray platelet syndrome	AR, pale platelets, splenomegaly
Paris-Trousseau thrombocytopenia	AD, cardiac defects, facial defects
Jacobsen syndrome	AD, congenital defects
ACTN1-related thrombocytopenia	AD, anizocytosis

AD – autosomal dominant; AR – autosomal recesive.

Immune Thrombocytopenia

The most common cause of thrombocytopenia is immune thrombocytopernia (ITP). Diagnosing ITP is diagnosis per exclusionem, there is no direct diagnostic test.

According to the International consensus report on the investigation and management of primary immune thrombocytopenia, the cornerstones of ITP diagnostics are as follows:

1 Patient's history
2 Physical examination
3 Peripheral blood count and smear with confirmation of thrombocytopenia to exclude pseudothrombocytopenia.

- Other procedures and tests recommended for ITP diagnostics are patient/family history, physical examination, reticulocyte count, quantitative immunoglobulin level analysis, blood group (Rh), direct antiglobulin test and serology for HIV and hepatitis C and evaluation of *Helicobacter pylori* infection [8, 9].

There are two forms of ITP:

Primary ITP

Autoimmune disease with isolated trombocytopenia (platelet count less than 100 x 10^9/L) and no other conditions, which can be associated with thrombocytopenia.

Secondary ITP

Immune mediated thrombocytopenia and other associated diseases (autoimmune diseases, lymphoproliferative diseases, infections). Systhemic lupus erytematosus (SLE) is an example of autoimmune disorder usually associated with thrombocytopenia. SLE_is a complex disease impairing various organs. About 15-25% of SLE patients present with thrombocytopenia, but only 5-10 % of them require therapy for this condition. Patient with SLE can also develop non-immune thrombocytopenias eg. thrombotic thrombocytopenic purpura, drug associated thrombocytopenia, antiphposfolipid antibody syndrom (both primary and secondary) and lupus vasculitis [10].

Some patients with malignant lymfoproliferative deseases e.g. Hodgkin´s lymphomas, and non-Hodgkin´s lymphomas can present with immune destruction of platelets. Immune platelet destruction is very common in patients with chronic lymfocytic leukemia (CLL). A second cause of thrombocytopenia in CLL is decreased production of platelets due to bone marrow infiltration by CLL cells.

Other factors can be also involved in thrombocytopenia in lymphoproliferative diseases - suppression of bone marrow by neoplastic cytokins and sequestration of platelets caused by splemomegaly [11]. Infection related thrombocytopenia.

Infection associated thrombocytopenia is common in childhood. Etiological agents are viruses e.g. cytomegalovirus, varicella, rubeola, mumps, Epstein-Barr virus, HHV-6 and HHV-8 viruses and HIV. *Helicobacter pylori* infection is associated with chronic ITP in many cases. In vitro studies showed cross reactivity of antibodies against *Helicobacter pylori* and platelet GpIIIA receptor. HIV-associated thrombocytopenia is present in 10% of patient with HIV positivity. Hepatitis C is another common cause of secondary ITP. Positivity of hepatitis infection is present in 10-36% patients with immune thrombocytopenia [12].

In primary ITP, bone marrow examination is recommended in patients older than 60 years of age, in those relapsing after remission, in patients not responding to first-line therapy, and in patients where splenectomy is considered.

ITP differential diagnosis is shown in Table 2.

Myelodysplastic Syndromes

Myelodysplastic syndromes (MDS) are a common cause of thrombocytopenia particularly in the elderly.

Recommendations for MDS diagnostics are as follows:

1 Peripheral blood smear and evaluation of dysplasia in one or more cell lines.
2 Bone marrow aspirate - evaluation of dysplasia in one or more hematopoietic cell lines.
3 Bone marrow biopsy - assessment of cellularity, fibrosis, megakaryocytes.
4 Cytogenetic analysis - detection of acquired clonal chromosomal abnormalities that can allow a conclusive diagnosis and also prognostic assessment.

Dysplastic changes in megakaryopoesis and thrombocytopenia can not only be signs of MDS, but also signs of idiopathic cytopenia of undetermined significance - megakaryocytycic dysplasia.

Table 2. Immune thrombocytopenia differential diagnosis

Immune thrombocytopenia (non ITP)	• Drug-associated thrombocytopenia • Heparin-induced thrombocytopenia • Neonatal alloimmune thrombocytopenia • Post-transfusion purpura
Non-immune thrombocytopenia	• Chronic alcohol abuse • Inherited thrombocytopenia • Thrombotic thrombocytopenic purpura • Thrombocytopenia due to sepsis • Disseminated intravascular coagulation • Kasabach-Merritt syndrome • Hypersplenism • Extracorporeal circulation
Bone marrow failure syndrome	• Aplastic anaemia, PNH • Myelodysplastic syndrome, AML • Amegakaryocytic thrombocytopenia
Coagulation disorder with thrombocytopenia	• von Willebrand disease type IIb • Platelet-type of von Willebrand disease
Secondary immune thrombocytopenias	• Autoimmune diseases • SLE • Rheumatoid arthritis • Felty's syndrome • Antiphospholipid antibody syndrome (ALPS) • Immune thyroid disease • Common variable immune deficiency • Chronic lymphocytic leukemia • Viral infection (hepatitis C, HIV, CMV) • *Helicobacter pylori* infection

References

[1] Cines, D. B., Bussel, J. B.: The ITP Syndrome: A diverse set of disorders with different immune mechanism. *Blood* 2009; 113: 6511-6521.

[2] British Committee for Standard in Haematology General Haematology Task Force Guidelines for the Investigation and Management of Idiopathic Thrombocytopenic Purpura (ITP) in adults, children and in pregnancy. *Br. J. Haematol.* 2003; 120: 574-596.

[3] Gernsheimer, G., James, A.: How I treat Thrombocytopenia in Pregnancy. *Blood* 2013; 121: 38-47.

[4] Rodeghiero, F., Stasi, R., Gernsheimer, T., et al.: Standardization of terminology, definitions and outcome criteria in immune thrombocytopenic purpura of adults and children: report from an international working group. *Blood* 2009; 113(11): 2386-2393.

[5] Balduini, C., Saviola, A.: Genetics of familial forms of thrombocytopenias. *Hum. Genet.* 2012 ;131: 1821-1832.

[6] Balduini, C., Pecci, A., Noris, P.: Diagnosis and management of inherited thrombocytopenias. *Semin. Throm. Hemost.* 2013; 39: 161-171.

[7] Albert, M. H., Bittner, T. C.: X-linked thrombocytopenia due to WAS mutations: clinical characteristic, ling-term outcome, and treatment options. *Blood* 2010; 115: 3231.

[8] Provan, D., Stasi, R., Newland, A. C., et al.: International consensus report on the investigation and management of primary immune thrombocytopenia. *Blood* 2010; 115 (2): 168-186.

[9] Neunert, C., Lim, W., Crowther, M., et al.: The American Society of Hematology 2011 evidence-based practice guideline for immune thrombocytopenia. *Blood*, 117(16): 4190-4207.

[10] Nossent, J. C., Swak, A. J.: Prevelence and significance of haemotological abnormalities in patients with systemic lupus erytematosus. *Q. J. Med.* 1991; 80: 605-612.

[11] Liebman, H. A.: Recognizing and treating secondary ITP associated with lymfoproliferative disorders. *Semin. Hematol.* 2009; 46: S33-S36.

[12] Liebman, H. A.: Viral–associated chronic immune thrombocytopenia. *Hematology* 2008; 212-218.

In: Thrombocytopenia
Editor: Mckenzie G. Bell

ISBN: 978-1-63321-713-3

Chapter 6

Heparin-Induced Thrombocytopenia: Current Concepts and Emerging Roles of Fondaparinux

Sumit Dahal, MBBS,[1] Smrity Upadhyay, MBBS,[2] Nabin Khanal, MBBS[2] and Vijaya Raj Bhatt, MBBS[3]*

[1]Institute of Medicine, Tribhuvan University,
Department of Medicine, Kathmandu, Nepal
[2]Creighton University Medical Center,
Department of Internal Medicine, Omaha, Nebraska, US
[3]University of Nebraska Medical Center, Department of Internal Medicine,
Division of Hematology-Oncology, Omaha, Nebraska, US

Abstract

Heparin induced thrombocytopenia (HIT) is a highly prothrombotic disorder mediated by platelet activating immunogloubulin G antibodies that bind to conformational epitopes on platelet factor 4 (PF4) when it is complexed with heparin. HIT occurs in 0.2% to 5% of adults treated with heparin. The risk is higher with the use of unfractionated heparin, longer duration of therapy, older women and surgical patients. HIT can present with isolated thrombocytopenia, thrombosis or other unusual manifestations. Typically, platelet count drops by ≥ 50% from baseline, beginning 5 to 10 days after the initiation of heparin therapy. However "rapid-onset" HIT and "delayed-onset" HIT can present diagnostic challenge. Approximately half of the untreated cases of isolated thrombocytopenia can develop thromboembolic events, predominantly venous thromboembolism. HIT is paradoxically under-recognized and over-diagnosed. As such, the current diagnostic algorithm utilizes both pre-test clinical probability and the results of laboratory assays. The widely utilized risk assessment system (4Ts score) provides an

* Correspondence: Vijaya Raj Bhatt, University of Nebraska Medical Center, Department of Internal Medicine, Division of Hematology-Oncology, 987680 Nebraska Medical Center, Omaha, NE 68198-7680, Phone: (402) 559-5388, Fax: (402) 559-6520, Email: vijaya.bhatt@unmc.edu

estimate of the pre-test probability of HIT by assigning scores based on the degree of thrombocytopenia, the timing of the drop in the platelet count, the presence of a thrombosis and the exclusion of other causes of thrombocytopenia. Laboratory diagnosis relies on the determination of the presence of circulating anti-PF4/heparin antibodies (immunologic assays) or the ability of such antibodies to cause platelet activation (functional assays). Enzyme linked immunosorbent assay has excellent sensitivity but suffers from poor specificity because of the detection of non-pathogenic anti-PF4/heparin antibodies. Functional assays such as serotonin release assay have significantly higher specificity but are not widely available. Treatment of HIT includes immediate withdrawal of all heparin products, initiation of a non-heparin anticoagulant (frequently argatroban) and transition to warfarin once the platelet count has normalized. Anticoagulation is maintained for at least 4 to 6 weeks in cases with isolated thrombocytopenia, and at least 3 months with thrombosis.

Subcutaneous fondaparinux has emerged as an alternative agent for the management of HIT. Multiple small case series have demonstrated comparable efficacy to argatroban and lepirudin, and excellent safety profile. Additionally, its fixed weight-based dosing and subcutaneous route prevents the need for frequent monitoring and allows easier transition to warfarin. Consequently, in the absence of kidney dysfunction, some experts utilize it as the therapy of choice in HIT. Conversely, there are documented cases of fondaparinux-associated HIT as well as worsening of HIT with the use of therapeutic fondaparinux. Although fondaparinux offers several advantages over alternate therapeutic options, such instances require carefulness during its use for the management of HIT.

Introduction

Heparin-induced thrombocytopenia (HIT), formerly HIT type II, is a highly prothrombotic disorder mediated by platelet-activating immunoglobulin G (IgG) antibodies that bind to conformational epitopes on platelet factor 4 (PF4) when it is complexed with polyanions (heparin) [1, 2]. HIT is reported to occur in 0.2% to 5% of adults treated with unfractionated heparin (UFH) [3], however, the incidence varies depending on the risk factors. There are an estimated 100,000 cases per year in the United States [4]. The devastating nature of the condition- with more than 35% of the untreated patients either dying or needing an amputation- makes it imperative to promptly recognize and manage the condition [5, 6]. HIT also places a significant economic burden on an individual patient as well as the healthcare system as a whole. On an average, a patient with HIT incurs a financial expenditure of more than $14,000 [7], whereas the total hospital cost per patient exceeds $100,000 [8].

Risk Factors

Risk factors for HIT can be categorized into heparin-related and host-related variables.

Heparin-related risk factors include type of heparin and duration of exposure. UFH is associated with a 5- to 10-fold higher risk of HIT than low molecular weight heparin (LMWH) [9]. In regards to the duration of therapy, the incidence of HIT is higher in patients receiving heparin for 6 or more days than those receiving it for shorter periods (2.6% vs 0.2%) [9, 10].

Host related factors include age, sex and patient population. HIT is rare in patients below the age of 40 years [11]. Females are at a greater risk of developing HIT with an odds ratio of 2.37 [12]. There is a 3-fold greater risk among surgical than medical patients [12]. Type of surgery is also important, with the incidence being the highest among patients who receive UFH after major orthopedic surgery. Although the rate of anti-PF4/heparin antibody formation is higher in patients undergoing cardiopulmonary bypass, the risk of HIT is lower than orthopedic surgery [13, 14]. Among the medical patients, those on hemodialysis or with an autoimmune disease, gout, or heart failure are at a greater risk of developing HIT [15]. While commonly encountered in patients newly initiated on hemodialysis (3.6%), it is rare in patients undergoing chronic intermittent hemodialysis (0.6%) despite repeated heparin exposure [16-18]. Unlike in low-density lipoprotein apheresis via dextran sulfate adsorption, the low incidence of HIT on long-term hemodialysis is not due to removal of PF4 from the plasma or the platelet surface [19, 20].

Pathogenesis

HIT is an idiosyncratic immune reaction characterized by the formation of IgG antibodies that recognize complexes of PF4 and polyanions, mainly heparin. PF4 is a chemokine synthesized during megakaryopoiesis and stored in platelet alpha-granules, and released in large amounts during platelet activation. PF4, which normally binds to glycosaminoglycans on the surfaces of endothelial cells, has a higher affinity for heparin compared to glycosaminoglycans. Hence, in the presence of circulating heparin, PF4 binds preferentially to heparin [21].

Formation of complexes of PF4 and heparin leads to the exposure of neoepitopes, which results in the formation of the anti-PF4/heparin antibodies. Anti-PF4/heparin IgG antibodies bind to heparin/PF4 complexes and the resultant ternary complexes bind to platelets through Fcγ receptor IIa expressed on the platelet surface [22]. Binding of antibody-antigen complexes to this receptor leads to increased platelet clearance, platelet activation, and release of procoagulant microparticles with activation of the coagulation cascade [23].

Anti-PF4/polyanion antibodies can also bind to platelet surface–bound PF4 in the absence of heparin and activate the platelets [24]. This results in so called "spontaneous HIT", characterized by the clinical and serological features of HIT in the absence of proximate heparin exposure [25]. This is common in the setting of sepsis where PF4 forms immunogenic complex with polyanions on the surface of bacteria [26]. Interaction of these complexes with monocytes, neutrophils, and endothelial cells via Fc receptors can contribute to thrombin generation seen in patients with HIT [23].

Although all patients with HIT have anti-PF4/heparin antibodies, most patients with anti-PF4/heparin antibodies do not have HIT. Systematic serosurveillance studies have shown that only a small proportion, at most 5% to 30% of patients who form anti-PF4/heparin antibodies, will develop clinical HIT [27, 28). What makes antibodies pathogenic is not known but may relate to the titer of the antibody or the size of the PF4–heparin complexes. UFH (3000 to 30,000 daltons) forms larger complexes with PF4 than LMWH (2000 to 9000 daltons). Fondaparinux (1728 daltons) is extremely unlikely to form complexes, which are large enough to cause platelet activation. Furthermore, certain conditions may predispose to the development of pathogenic anti-PF4/heparin antibodies. This is illustrated by the finding that heparin use in coronary artery bypass surgery results in anti-PF4/heparin antibodies formation in 20 to 50% but HIT in only about 1% of patients. Conversely, heparin use in orthopedic surgery leads to the development of anti-PF4/heparin antibodies in about 10% of patients and HIT in about 5% [14].

The HIT immune response wanes over time. Functional assays become negative at a median of 50 days after heparin cessation, whereas anti-PF4/heparin antibody titers decline more slowly and are no longer detectable in 60% of patients by day 100 [29].

There is growing interest in the possible role of B-cell tolerance in the pathogenesis of HIT [30]. Glycosaminoglycan and non-glycosaminoglycan polyanionic macromolecules such as DNA and RNA continually interact with and produce structural modifications in PF4, making them immunogenic [31, 32]. B-cell tolerance to epitopes recognized by HIT antibodies is established early in life and plays a critical role in controlling production of anti-PF4/polyanion antibodies [30]. This B-cell anergy also explains why only a small fraction of patients exposed to heparin experience HIT. Breakdown of this tolerance, such as with an inflammatory stimulus, can lead to anti-PF4/heparin antibody production [30]. This may explain increased incidence of HIT antibodies and clinical HIT with heparin exposure during cardiopulmonary bypass or orthopedic surgery- procedures associated with inflammatory milieu secondary to tissue trauma [30, 33]. This tolerance breakdown concept is also consistent with the atypical immune response seen in HIT – production of IgG class of antibodies when exposed to heparin for the first time, and the rapid production and loss of anti-PF4/heparin antibodies [29, 30, 34].

Clinical Features

The clinical features of HIT can be protean, including isolated thrombocytopenia, thrombosis and other unusual manifestations.

Thrombocytopenia

Typically, the drop in the platelet count begins 5 to 10 days after the initiation of heparin therapy in heparin-naïve individuals. Patients exposed to heparin in past 3 months and particularly within past 30 days can develop thrombocytopenia more rapidly ("rapid-onset" HIT) [29]. Rarely, manifestations of HIT may develop after heparin is discontinued. This phenomenon, referred to as "delayed-onset" HIT, occurs at a median of 10 to 14 days after heparin withdrawal and is often associated with disseminated intravascular coagulation (DIC) [35].

The platelet count frequently falls by $\geq$ 50% from baseline, and the typical median nadir platelet count is in the range of 60 $\times 10^9$/L. The absolute platelet count seldom falls below 20 $\times$ 10^9/L in the absence of concomitant DIC [36].

Thrombosis

About half of all the patients with HIT present with a new thromboembolic complication, referred to as "HIT with thrombosis" (HIT-T). Of those patients presenting with isolated thrombocytopenia, almost half will subsequently develop a thromboembolic event if left untreated. Venous thromboembolism is four times more common than arterial thromboembolic events [5]. In addition to deep venous thrombosis, pulmonary embolism is also common. Arterial thrombosis most commonly involves the arteries of the lower limbs, with thrombotic strokes and myocardial infarction seen less frequently [37]. Other rare thrombotic events include cerebral sinus venous thrombosis and adrenal vein thrombosis [23].

Spontaneous Bleeding

In contrast to most other cases of drug-induced thrombocytopenia, significant bleeding is rare, even with severe thrombocytopenia. In prospective studies, bleeding complications were not significantly increased in HIT patients over non-thrombocytopenic controls [38). In fact, the presence of petechiae or hemorrhage is frequently considered as evidence against the diagnosis of HIT.

Unusual Manifestations

Anaphylactoid reactions after intravenous heparin bolus, skin necrosis at injection sites and transient global amnesia are some of the unusual manifestations seen with HIT [39].

Diagnosis

The complexity of making a diagnosis of HIT is reflected by the fact that HIT is paradoxically under-recognized and over-diagnosed depending on a clinical scenario. Patients, who develop HIT, often have alternate causes of thrombocytopenia. Hence, in the absence of a high index of suspicion for HIT, the diagnosis may be missed. Conversely, overuse of serological tests, which frequently demonstrate non-pathogenic anti-PF4/heparin antibodies, may lead to over-diagnosis of HIT.

The current diagnostic algorithm for HIT, therefore, utilizes both pre-test clinical probability and the results of laboratory assays.

Clinical Diagnosis

Clinical features that may favor a diagnosis of HIT

1. Fall in platelet count begins 5-10 days after heparin exposure
2. Fall in platelet count $\geq$ 50%

3. Nadir platelet count ≥ 20 x 10^9/L
4. Thrombosis
5. Unusual manifestations: Skin necrosis at subcutaneous heparin injection sites; anaphylactoid reactions after intravenous heparin bolus; transient global amnesia
6. Absence of petechiae and significant bleeding
7. Absence of other causes of thrombocytopenia such as infection or drugs other than heparin

Clinical Scoring Models

Several clinical scoring systems have been developed to calculate a pre-test probability of HIT. The widely utilized "4Ts" score provides an estimate of pre-test probability of HIT by assigning scores based on the degree of thrombocytopenia, the timing of thrombocytopenia, the presence of a thrombosis, and the presence of alternate cause (table 1) [40, 41]. The pre-test probability of HIT is considered high for a score of 6-8, intermediate for a score of 4-5, and low for a score of 0-3. This 4Ts scoring system has a high negative predictive value but a low positive predictive value, thus making it more useful in ruling out the diagnosis of HIT. It, however, suffers from a modest inter-observer agreement. The HIT Expert Probability score [42], a newer scoring system, has greater inter-observer agreement and correlation with the diagnosis of HIT. However it has not undergone prospective validation. On retrospective comparison, there was no significant difference in performance of the HIT Expert Probability score and 4Ts score [43].

Table 1. Pretest clinical scoring system for heparin-induced thrombocytopenia

Findings	2 points	1 point	0 point
Thrombocytopenia	>50% platelet drop from baseline with a platelet nadir ≥20 x 10^9/L	30%-50% platelet drop from baseline, or platelet nadir 10-19 x 10^9/L	<30% platelet drop from baseline or platelet nadir < 10 x 10^9/L
Timing of the decline in platelet count	5 to 10 days; or within 1 day in patients with heparin exposure in past 30 days	After day 10; or within 1 day with heparin exposure in past 31-100 days	Within 4 days with no recent heparin exposure
Thrombosis or other sequelae	Proven thrombosis, skin necrosis, or acute systemic reaction after heparin bolus.	Progressive, recurrent or suspected thrombosis; non-necrotizing erythematous skin lesions	None
Alternate cause of thrombocytopenia	None	Possible	Definite

Source: [40], adapted with permission from the publisher. Copyright: 2006, John Wiley and Sons.

To estimate the probability of HIT in patients following cardiopulmonary bypass, Lillo Le Louët score has been designed [44]. However an independent study showed this score to have a low negative predictive value, suggesting inadequate sensitivity for its use as a clinical screening test [45].

Laboratory Diagnosis

Laboratory diagnosis relies on the determination of the presence of circulating anti-PF4/heparin antibodies (immunologic assays) or the ability of such antibodies to cause platelet activation (functional assays).

Immunologic Assays

The most widely used immunologic assay, polyspecific solid-phase enzyme-linked immunosorbent assay (ELISA), offers an ease of performance, rapid turnaround time and high sensitivity (> 95%) with excellent negative predictive value [46]. The limitation of the test includes poor specificity (50% to 89%) because of the detection of non-pathogenic anti-PF4/heparin antibodies [46]. Utilization of IgG-specific ELISA and measurement of antibody titers (optical density) can improve the specificity of the test. Optical density is directly associated with the 4Ts score and HIT Expert Probability score, risk of thrombosis and the likelihood of a positive functional assay [42, 47]. With an optical density of 0.40 to < 1.00, the probability of strong positive functional assay, and hence HIT, is ≤5%. An optical density of > 1.00 is strongly correlated with pathologic antibodies. The probability of a strong positive functional assay and HIT reaches around 90% with an optical density of > 2.00 [47].

High-dose heparin confirmatory procedure, in which inhibition of a positive ELISA test by ≥50% in the presence of excess heparin, is regarded as a confirmatory test for detection of heparin-dependent antibodies. This additional test also improves the specificity of ELISA [48]. Similarly, competitive ELISA using KKO, a HIT-like murine monoclonal anti-PF4/heparin IgG, has been developed to enable distinction of potentially pathogenic antibodies form nonpathogenic antibodies [49]. The pathogenic antibodies inhibit binding of KKO to PF4/heparin complexes, whereas non-pathogenic antibodies do not. This is based on a recent observation that pathogenic and nonpathogenic antibodies bind to different epitopes on PF4/heparin complexes [50].

Particle gel and magnetic particle chemiluminescent immunoassays, which permit the detection of anti-PF4/heparin antibodies within minutes, as opposed to the hours required for ELISA-based tests, have been developed [51, 52]. However, efforts to detect PF4/heparin-specific memory B cells using modified enzyme-linked immunosorbent spot (ELISPOT) assay, thus far, have been unsuccessful [53].

Functional Assays

^{14}C-serotonin release assay and heparin-induced platelet activation assay, the two most extensively studied functional tests, have significantly higher specificity than immunologic assays, and are frequently used for disease confirmation [54, 55]. Serotonin release assay measures the release of ^{14}C-serotonin from activated platelets, whereas heparin-induced platelet activation assay utilizes platelet aggregation as its endpoint. These tests, which are technically demanding and require the use of radioisotope (in case of serotonin release assay) and fresh donor platelets, have long turnaround times and are not widely available [56].

Other functional assays with potential use in HIT include a whole-blood impedance aggregometry assay, and flow cytometry-based assays that detect platelet microparticles, P-selectin expression, and annexin V binding [57-60]. A novel functional assay, utilizing a chicken B-lymphocyte line transfected with the human Fcγ receptor IIa coupled to a luciferase reporter, offers increased feasibility (as it uses a cell-line that can be stored and retrieved as needed instead of fresh platelets, and measures light emission rather than radioactivity or platelet aggregation as an endpoint for cellular activation) [61]. However, prospective evaluation in a larger cohort of patients is needed to confirm the utility of this assay.

Approach to Diagnosis

Thrombocytopenic patients with low clinical probability require no further evaluation for HIT. Patients with intermediate or high clinical probability should undergo ELISA test. A weakly positive ELISA (optical density 0.40–0.99) in patients with intermediate clinical probability is unlikely to be HIT and requires no further evaluation. In patients with weakly positive ELISA (optical density 0.40–0.99) and high clinical probability, and those with moderately or strongly positive ELISA (optical density≥1.00), functional assays may be obtained for confirmation [3].

Treatment

A diagnosis or suspicion of HIT warrants immediate withdrawal of all heparin products, including heparin-containing flushes and catheters. Additionally, nonheparin anticoagulant should be promptly initiated [62]. Several parenteral anticoagulants are available for the treatment of HIT including direct thrombin inhibitors such as argatroban, lepirudin and bivalirudin; and indirect factor X inhibitors such as danaparoid and fondaparinux (table 2).

Transitioning to Oral Anticoagulation

Early introduction of vitamin K antagonists (such as warfarin) should be avoided, since this has the potential to worsen the prothrombotic state through a rapid reduction in protein C and S (natural anticoagulants) [63]. Once the platelet count has returned to a normal level after an acute episode of HIT, warfarin should be introduced, and overlapped with a non-heparin anticoagulant for a minimum of 5 days [62].

Table 2. Parenteral non-heparin anticoagulants used in heparin-induced thrombocytopenia

Agent	Indication/ Availability	Pharmacology*	Side effects
Direct Thrombin Inhibitors			
Argatroban	FDA approved for the treatment of HIT.	It has hepatobiliary clearance, immediate onset of action and achieves a steady-state anticoagulant effect within 1 to 3 hours. Dosing: Normal organ function: 2 μg/kg/min Liver dysfunction, heart failure, post cardiac surgery, anasarca: 0.5-1.2 μg/kg per minute	Hemorrhage, chest pain, hypotension, cough, and vomiting. Rebound hypercoagulability if discontinued before resolution of a procoagulant state (104).
Lepirudin	FDA approved for the treatment of HIT but no longer manufactured.	It has renal clearance with a half-life of 80 minutes. Dosing: Bolus: 0.2 mg/kg (only for life- or limb-threatening thrombosis) Continuous infusion: 0.10 to 0.005 mg/kg/hour depending on blood creatinine level	Hemorrhage, bronchospasm, rash, and edema. Formation of antilepirudin antibodies (~50% of cases) (105), which may potentiate its anticoagulant activity necessitating a dose reduction.
Bivalirudin	FDA approved for HIT patients undergoing percutaneous cardiac intervention.†	It undergoes renal and enzymatic clearance, and has a brief half-life of 25 minutes which allows for rapid dose titration. Dosing: Normal organ function: 0.15 mg/kg/hour Renal or hepatic dysfunction: dose reduction	Hemorrhage, back pain, hypotension, headache and vomiting.
Indirect Factor Xa inhibitors			
Danaparoid	Available outside US but not in the United States.	It has renal clearance and a long half-life (24 hours). Dosing Bolus: 1500 U for <60 kg, 2250 U for 60-75 kg; 3000 U for 75-90 kg; and 3750 U for >90 kg Accelerated initial infusion: 400 U/hour x 4 hours, then 300 U/hour x 4 hours Maintenance infusion: Normal renal function: 200 U/hour Renal insufficiency: 150 U/hour	Hemorrhage. Potential for cross-reactivity with anti-PF4/heparin antibodies.
Fondaparinux	Not approved for HIT	It has renal clearance and a long half-life (17-20 hours). Dosing < 50 kg: 5 mg subcutaneously daily 50-100 kg: 7.5 mg subcutaneously daily > 100 kg: 10 mg subcutaneously daily Cl_{Cr} 30-50 mL/min: use caution Cl_{Cr} < 30 mL/min: contraindicated.	Hemorrhage including rare instances of epidural/spinal hematoma, pruritus and rash. Additional details in the text and table 3.

Source: Multiple references including (3) for pharmacology column.

Cr indicates serum creatinine; and Cl_{Cr}, creatinine clearance.

*Argatroban, lepirudin, and bivalirudin are monitored using aPTT with a goal of 1.5-3.0 times patients' baseline. Danaparoid is monitored using anti-factor Xa with a goal of 0.5-0.8 U/ml. Fondaparinux does not require routine monitoring, but anti-factor Xa may be utilized for monitoring (3).

†Bivalirudin has been utilized successfully in cardiac surgery.

Transferring to warfarin, however, may be more complicated than simply achieving a therapeutic international normalized ratio (INR) since the parental anticoagulants such as argatroban can also increase INR. Neglecting this effect can cause inadequate anti-coagulation once the patient is switched to warfarin alone. Hence, a trial to stop the parental anticoagulant is required, as described below. Argatroban is stopped when INR of > 4 is reached on combined anticoagulation with warfarin and argatroban dose of ≤2 μg/kg per minute. Then, a repeat INR is obtained in 4-6 hours. If INR returns to be <2, argatroban is resumed at 10% increased dose, and the procedure is repeated until INR ≥2 is achieved off argatroban. For argatroban initially being used at a dose of >2 μg/kg per minute, the dose is first reduced to ≤2 μg/kg per minute, followed by the above algorithm [3, 64].

Duration of Anticoagulation

The risk of thrombosis, although reversible, persists for 4 to 6 weeks. Hence, the duration of anticoagulation should be at least 4 to 6 weeks in HIT patients with isolated thrombocytopenia [5, 62], and at least 3 months or longer, as indicated, in HIT with thrombosis.

Platelet Transfusion

HIT generally does not present with a bleeding manifestation; therefore, platelet transfusion is rarely necessary. However platelet transfusion in clinically indicated patients with suspected or confirmed HIT may cause appropriate increment in the platelet count and cessation of bleeding in the majority, and may not be associated with increased thrombotic complication [65]. Hence, platelet transfusion in the setting of HIT is most likely safe and effective, and should not be withheld in bleeding patients [65, 66].

Heparin Re-Exposure for Cardiovascular Procedures

Heparin is a preferred intraoperative anticoagulant during cardiac and vascular surgery because of its favorable pharmacokinetics, easy monitoring, and reversibility with protamine [3]. The risk of recurrent HIT in patients with a previous history of HIT, who receive subsequent re-exposure to heparin, is generally low [67-69]. The risk remains low even if anti-PF4/heparin antibodies persist at the time of re-exposure, as long as there are no platelet-activating antibodies [69]. Since the antibody formation do not occur any quicker on re-exposure and take a median of 5-7 days, limiting heparin use for intraoperative anticoagulation may minimize the risk of HIT [69]. However, postoperative anticoagulation, if needed, should be achieved with alternative anticoagulants.

ELISA and functional assay should be tested before considering heparin reuse. For invasive cardiovascular procedures, heparin may be used for intraoperative anticoagulation in cases with remote HIT (negative immunologic and functional assays) [67]. In cases with a negative functional assay and a positive ELISA, surgery should be delayed; if surgery cannot be delayed, heparin may be used with caution [70]. In cases with a positive functional assay, the surgery should be delayed; if surgery cannot be delayed, an alternative anticoagulant such as bivalirudin should be used. However for percutaneous vascular procedures, bivalirudin is recommended over heparin in all patients with a history of HIT [3].

Fondaparinux and HIT

Fondaparinux is a synthetic pentasaccharide that strongly binds to antithrombin, causing prolonged inhibition of activated factor X, but not thrombin [71].

Fondaparinux as the Treatment of HIT

It has been shown to be safe and effective in a large variety of clinical settings of antithrombotic prophylaxis and treatment. Even though not recommended by manufacturer or regulatory bodies, fondaparinux is routinely utilized in clinical practice by some experts as the therapy of choice in HIT patients with normal renal function (table 3) [2, 72, 73].

Table 3. Safety and efficacy of fondaparinux use in heparin-induced thrombocytopenia

Study	Number of patients	Agents	Major Bleeding	New Thrombosis	Remarks
Lobo, 2008 (106)*	17	Fondaparinux vs. Lepirudin/Argatroban	0	0	Amputation 14% vs. 10%, but death 0 vs. 20%
Grouzi, 2010 (107)	44	Fondaparinux vs. Lepirudin	0	0	Death 4% vs. 10%
Warkentin, 2011 (108)	16	Fondaparinux	6%	0	
Goldfarb, 2011 (109)	8	Fondaparinux	0	0	
Bhatt, 2013 (77)	8	Fondaparinux	--	--	8 cases of fondaparinux-associated HIT (confirmed or suspected)
Bhatt, 2013 (79)	3	Fondaparinux	--	--	Worsening of thrombosis or thrombocytopenia in 100% cases
Cegarra-Sanmartin, 2014 (110)	15	Fondaparinux	13%	0	Cardiac patients with renal failure in 12 patients

*This study included a prospective cohort of fondaparinux treated patients; however, lepirudin/argatroban cohort in this study and the cohorts in other studies were retrospective cohorts.

Benken, 2014 (111) demonstrated 12% overt bleeding and 37% thrombotic events with use of fondaparinux in 8 patients with suspected or confirmed HIT, who had underwent left ventricular assist device. However, the majority of these patients had low-moderate HIT score and low optical density of anti-PF4/HIT antibodies on ELISA, thus suggesting that many of these patients may not have had HIT.

It has also been used as a preferred therapy in patients with a history of HIT [74, 75], as a bridge between intravenous non-heparin anticoagulant and warfarin, or as an alternate therapy to warfarin after recovery of the platelet count (e.g. in pregnancy or warfarin-associated skin necrosis) [74].

Advantages of fondaparinux over direct thrombin inhibitors:

1. Its long half life (~17-20 hours) achieves stable level of anticoagulation and may reduce the risk of rebound hypercoagulability with abrupt drug cessation.
2. No interference with the protein C pathway
3. Very low intra- and inter-subject variability allows fixed weight-based dosing. When needed, drug levels can be measured reliably using anti-factor Xa assays (conversely, activated partial thromboplastin time monitoring for direct thrombin inhibitors can be unreliable in DIC or liver disease).
4. The lack of interference of fondaparinux on INR may make subsequent overlapping therapy with warfarin easier to manage (conversely, direct thrombin inhibitors, especially argatroban, can raise the INR, thus complicating the assessment of the effects of warfarin).
5. It also has lower daily cost than most direct thrombin inhibitors [73].

Fondaparinux as the Cause of HIT

There is dissociation in fondaparinux immunogenicity and cross-reactivity. Anti-PF4/heparin antibodies are generated as frequently in patients receiving fondaparinux as those with LMWH, however, fondaparinux generally does not promote binding of these antibodies to PF4 or platelet activation [76, 77].

Recently, several cases of possible association of fondaparinux with HIT and its failure in HIT patients have been reported [77-86]. The development of fondaparinux-associated HIT is rare but can occur in the setting of a pro-inflammatory state, prior HIT, or an exposure with UFH or LMWH. Patients with fondaparinux-associated HIT present with the usual clinical manifestations. Almost one fourth of the patients also have bilateral adrenal hemorrhage or infarct [77].

The presence of intermediate to high 4T score and positive functional assays are generally adequate for diagnosing fondaparinux-associated HIT. However, demonstration of fondaparinux-dependent platelet activation is necessary in cases with recent heparin exposure [77].

While the off-label use of fondaparinux in HIT is increasingly common owing to its ease of use, safety and efficacy, the fondaparinux data are derived from small observational studies. The limited experience with fondaparinux use in HIT, risk of fondaparinux-associated HIT, albeit small, and documented cases of fondaparinux failure mandate carefulness during its use for the management of HIT [77, 79].

Experimental Treatments in HIT

Parenteral direct thrombin inhibitors such as argatroban and lepirudin have long been the mainstay of HIT treatment, and will likely continue to be the treatment of choice for acute HIT with thrombosis. However they require frequent monitoring, cause serious bleeding and are expensive [62, 87]. With two of the commonly employed parenteral agents – lepirudin and danaparoid – no more available in US, the need for newer agents effective in HIT has increased. Moreover, the long-term anticoagulation with warfarin for the prevention and extended treatment of HIT is also fraught with problems. Apart from the unpredictable pharmacokinetics and the need for routine monitoring, warfarin has slow onset of action and the potential to precipitate venous limb gangrene or skin necrosis, which are of particular concern when treating a highly hypercoagulable condition such as HIT. Given that less than 10% of patients suspected of having HIT actually have the disorder, the search is for anticoagulant regimens that are safe with low risk of bleeding, effective for both HIT and non-HIT thrombosis and allow easy or no monitoring [87, 88]. In this context, the orally active direct thrombin inhibitor, dabigatran, and factor Xa inhibitors such as rivaroxaban and apixaban hold promise [71, 72, 74, 89-93]. Co-administration of a low sulfated heparin, 2-O, 3-O desulfated heparin, with heparin may reduce the immunogenicity of heparin and hence, the development of HIT [90] but this remains to be confirmed.

The pharmacological properties of the following agents offer attractive therapeutic options for HIT, however, these agents are investigational and should not be used in HIT outside of a clinical trial.

Dabigatran

It is an oral reversible direct thrombin inhibitor. It has been approved for the prevention of stroke in patients with atrial fibrillation. It does not need monitoring, has rapid peak blood levels and does not interact with PF4, making it suitable for the prevention and treatment of HIT, especially in patients with a history of HIT who require anticoagulation (89-91).

Rivaroxaban

It is an oral direct factor Xa inhibitor. It does not cross-react with HIT antibodies, mobilize PF4 from platelets or interact with PF4 [90, 93]. Moreover, unlike fondaparinux, it also blocks the release of PF4 from activated platelets [93]. A phase 3 clinical trial (http://ClinicalTrials.gov number, NCT01598168) is currently underway to validate the role of rivaroxaban in HIT.

Apixaban

It is an oral direct factor Xa inhibitor that has recently been approved for the prevention of stroke and systemic embolism in patients with AF. It does not cross react with HIT antibodies or cause platelet activation and aggregation, and may provide an option for the long-term management and prevention of HIT [92].

2-O, 3-O Desulfated Heparin

It is derived from UFH heparin by desulfation at the 2-O and 3-O position and lacks most of the anticoagulant effects of UFH. It may prevent formation of immunogenic PF4/heparin complexes. When it is given together with heparin, it may have the potential to reduce the development of HIT [90].

Therapeutic Plasma Exchange

Plasma exchange lowers the HIT antibody level acutely, but the effect is usually transient (94). It has been used successfully for temporary reduction of HIT antibody titer prior to cardiopulmonary bypass in patients, who require heparin re-exposure, as well as for treatment of established HIT [95-101]. Plasma exchange is most effective when used early in the disease, preferably within the first four days [102].

Prevention

Use of subcutaneous LMWH instead of intravenous UFH can reduce the incidence of HIT. Monitoring of the platelet count during heparin therapy has been recommended when the risk of HIT is greater than 1% (e.g., in postoperative patients receiving prophylactic or therapeutic UFH; or in patients receiving either UFH or LMWH after a cardiac surgery) [103].

Conclusion

HIT is a rare but potentially catastrophic complication of heparin therapy. Over the years, our understanding of this condition has greatly increased with a well-elucidated pathogenesis and clinical profile. Prompt diagnosis using a combination of clinical pretest score and laboratory assays, and early initiation of appropriate anticoagulation can significantly decrease the morbidity and mortality associated with HIT. With newer diagnostic and treatment modalities in pipeline, we can expect significant changes in the way we approach this condition in the near future.

Conflict of Interest/Financial support: None.

References

[1] Amiral J, Bridey F, Dreyfus M, Vissac A, Fressinaud E, Wolf M, et al. Platelet factor 4 complexes to heparin is the target for antibodies generated in heparin-induced thrombocytopenia. *Thromb Haemost*. 1992;68(1):95-6.

[2] Kelton JG, Arnold DM, Bates SM. Nonheparin anticoagulants for heparin-induced thrombocytopenia. *The New England journal of medicine*. 2013 Feb 21;368(8):737-44.

[3] Cuker A, Cines DB. How I treat heparin-induced thrombocytopenia. *Blood*. 2012 Mar 8;119(10):2209-18.

[4] Shuster TA, Silliman WR, Coats RD, Mureebe L, Silver D. Heparin-induced thrombocytopenia: twenty-nine years later. *J. Vasc. Surg*. 2003;38(6):1316-22.

[5] Warkentin TE, Kelton JG. A 14-year study of heparin-induced thrombocytopenia. *The American journal of medicine*. 1996;101(5):502-7.

[6] Wallis DE, Workman DL, Lewis BE, Steen L, Pifarre R, Moran JF. Failure of early heparin cessation as treatment for heparin-induced thrombocytopenia. *The American journal of medicine*. 1999;106(6):629-35.

[7] Smythe MA, Koerber JM, Fitzgerald M, Mattson JC. The financial impact of heparin-induced thrombocytopenia. *Chest*. 2008 Sep;134(3):568-73.

[8] Baroletti S, Piovella C, Fanikos J, Labreche M, Lin J, Goldhaber SZ. Heparin-induced thrombocytopenia (HIT): clinical and economic outcomes. *Thromb Haemost.* 2008 Dec;100(6):1130-5.

[9] Martel N, Lee J, Wells PS. Risk for heparin-induced thrombocytopenia with unfractionated and low-molecular-weight heparin thromboprophylaxis: a meta-analysis. *Blood.* 2005;106(8):2710-5.

[10] Smythe MA, Koerber JM, Mattson JC. The incidence of recognized heparin-induced thrombocytopenia in a large, tertiary care teaching hospital. *CHEST Journal.* 2007;131(6):1644-9.

[11] Stein PD, Hull RD, Matta F, Yaekoub AY, Liang J. Incidence of thrombocytopenia in hospitalized patients with venous thromboembolism. *The American journal of medicine.* 2009;122(10):919-30.

[12] Warkentin TE, Sheppard J-AI, Sigouin CS, Kohlmann T, Eichler P, Greinacher A. Gender imbalance and risk factor interactions in heparin-induced thrombocytopenia. *Blood.* 2006;108(9):2937-41.

[13] Bauer TL, Arepally G, Konkle BA, Mestichelli B, Shapiro SS, Cines DB, et al. Prevalence of heparin-associated antibodies without thrombosis in patients undergoing cardiopulmonary bypass surgery. *Circulation.* 1997;95(5):1242-6.

[14] Warkentin TE, Sheppard J-AI, Horsewood P, Simpson PJ, Moore JC, Kelton JG. Impact of the patient population on the risk for heparin-induced thrombocytopenia. *Blood.* 2000;96(5):1703-8.

[15] Kato S, Takahashi K, Ayabe K, Samad R, Fukaya E, Friedmann P, et al. Heparin-induced thrombocytopenia: analysis of risk factors in medical inpatients. *Br. J. Haematol.* 2011 Aug;154(3):373-7.

[16] Luzzatto G, Bertoli M, Cella G, Fabris F, Zaia B, Girolami A. Platelet count, anti-heparin/platelet factor 4 antibodies and tissue factor pathway inhibitor plasma antigen level in chronic dialysis. *Thromb Res.* 1998;89(3):115-22.

[17] Yamamoto S, Koide M, Matsuo M, Suzuki S, Ohtaka M, Saika S, et al. Heparin-induced thrombocytopenia in hemodialysis patients. *Am. J. Kidney Dis.* 1996;28(1):82-5.

[18] Matsuo T, Kobayashi H, Matsuo M, Wanaka K, Nakamoto H, Matsushima H, et al. Frequency of anti-heparin-PF4 complex antibodies (HIT antibodies) in uremic patients on chronic intermittent hemodialysis. *Pathophysiol. Haemost Thromb.* 2009;35(6):445-50.

[19] Tanhehco YC, Cuker A, Rudnick M, Sachais BS. Investigation of a potential protective mechanism against heparin-induced thrombocytopenia in patients on chronic intermittent hemodialysis. *Thromb Res.* 2013 Mar;131(3):244-8.

[20] Tanhehco YC, Rux AH, Sachais BS. Low-density lipoprotein apheresis reduces platelet factor 4 on the surface of platelets: a possible protective mechanism against heparin-induced thrombocytopenia and thrombosis. *Transfusion* (Paris). 2011 May;51(5):1022-9.

[21] Cines DB, Rauova L, Arepally G, Reilly MP, McKenzie SE, Sachais BS, et al. Heparin-induced thrombocytopenia: An autoimmune disorder regulated through dynamic autoantigen assembly/disassembly. *J. Clin. Apher.* 2007;22(1):31-6.

[22] Visentin GP, Ford SE, Scott JP, Aster RH. Antibodies from patients with heparin-induced thrombocytopenia/thrombosis are specific for platelet factor 4 complexed with heparin or bound to endothelial cells. *J. Clin. Invest.* 1994;93(1):81.

[23] Warkentin TE. Heparin-induced thrombocytopenia: pathogenesis and management. *Br. J. Haematol.* 2003;121(4):535-55.

[24] Rauova L, Zhai L, Kowalska MA, Arepally GM, Cines DB, Poncz M. Role of platelet surface PF4 antigenic complexes in heparin-induced thrombocytopenia pathogenesis: diagnostic and therapeutic implications. *Blood.* 2006;107(6):2346-53.

[25] Warkentin TE, Basciano PA, Knopman J, Bernstein RA. Spontaneous heparin-induced thrombocytopenia syndrome: two new cases and a proposal for defining this disorder. *Blood.* 2014 Mar 27.

[26] Greinacher A, Holtfreter B, Krauel K, Gätke D, Weber C, Ittermann T, et al. Association of natural anti-platelet factor 4/heparin antibodies with periodontal disease. *Blood.* 2011;118(5):1395-401.

[27] Amiral J, Bridey F, Wolf M, Boyer-Neumann C, Fressinaud E, Vissac A, et al. Antibodies to macromolecular platelet factor 4-heparin complexes in heparin-induced thrombocytopenia: a study of 44 cases. *Thromb Haemost.* 1995;73(1):21-8.

[28] Warkentin TE, Sheppard J-AI, Moore JC, Moore KM, Sigouin CS, Kelton JG. Laboratory testing for the antibodies that cause heparin-induced thrombocytopenia: how much class do we need? *J. Lab. Clin. Med.* 2005;146(6):341-6.

[29] Warkentin TE, Kelton JG. Temporal aspects of heparin-induced thrombocytopenia. *N. Engl. J. Med.* 2001;344(17):1286-92.

[30] Zheng Y, Wang AW, Yu M, Padmanabhan A, Tourdot BE, Newman DK, et al. B-cell tolerance regulates production of antibodies causing heparin-induced thrombocytopenia. *Blood.* 2014 Feb 6;123(6):931-4.

[31] Visentin GP, Moghaddam M, Beery SE, McFarland JG, Aster RH. Heparin is not required for detection of antibodies associated with heparin-induced thrombocytopenia/thrombosis. *J. Lab. Clin. Med.* 2001;138(1):22-31.

[32] Jaax ME, Krauel K, Marschall T, Brandt S, Gansler J, Fürll B, et al. Complex formation with nucleic acids and aptamers alters the antigenic properties of platelet factor 4. *Blood.* 2013;122(2):272-81.

[33] Lubenow N, Hinz P, Thomaschewski S, Lietz T, Vogler M, Ladwig A, et al. The severity of trauma determines the immune response to PF4/heparin and the frequency of heparin-induced thrombocytopenia. *Blood.* 2010;115(9):1797-803.

[34] Warkentin TE, Sheppard J-AI, Moore JC, Cook RJ, Kelton JG. Studies of the immune response in heparin-induced thrombocytopenia. *Blood.* 2009;113(20):4963-9.

[35] Warkentin TE, Kelton JG. Delayed-onset heparin-induced thrombocytopenia and thrombosis. *Ann. Intern. Med.* 2001;135(7):502-6.

[36] Warkentin TE, editor. Clinical presentation of heparin-induced thrombocytopenia. Semin Hematol; 1998.

[37] Greinacher A, Farner B, Kroll H, Kohlmann T, Warkentin TE, Eichler P. Clinical features of heparin-induced thrombocytopenia including risk factors for thrombosis. *Thromb Haemost.* 2005;94:132-5.

[38] Warkentin TE, Levine MN, Hirsh J, Horsewood P, Roberts RS, Gent M, et al. Heparin-induced thrombocytopenia in patients treated with low-molecular-weight heparin or unfractionated heparin. *N. Engl. J. Med.* 1995;332(20):1330-6.

[39] Warkentin TE, Roberts RS, Hirsh J, Kelton JG. Heparin-Induced Skin Lesions and Other Unusual Sequelae of the Heparin-Induced Thrombocytopenia Syndrome A Nested Cohort Study. *Chest.* 2005;127(5):1857-61.

[40] Lo G, Juhl D, Warkentin T, Sigouin C, Eichler P, Greinacher A. Evaluation of pretest clinical score (4 T's) for the diagnosis of heparin-induced thrombocytopenia in two clinical settings. *J. Thromb Haemost.* 2006;4(4):759-65.

[41] Warkentin TE, Heddle NM. Laboratory diagnosis of immune heparin-induced thrombocytopenia. *Curr. Hematol. Rep.* 2003 Mar;2(2):148-57.

[42] Cuker A, Arepally G, Crowther MA, Rice L, Datko F, Hook K, et al. The HIT Expert Probability (HEP) Score: a novel pre-test probability model for heparin-induced thrombocytopenia based on broad expert opinion. *J. Thromb. Haemost.* 2010 Dec;8(12):2642-50.

[43] Uaprasert N, Chanswangphuwana C, Akkawat B, Rojnuckarin P. Comparison of diagnostic performance of the heparin-induced thrombocytopenia expert probability and the 4Ts score in screening for heparin-induced thrombocytopenia. *Blood Coagul Fibrinolysis.* 2013;24(3):261-8.

[44] Louet LL, Boutouyrie P, Alhenc-Gelas M, Le Beller C, Gautier I, Aiach M, et al. Diagnostic score for heparin-induced thrombocytopenia after cardiopulmonary bypass. *J. Thromb Haemost.* 2004;2(11):1882-8.

[45] Piednoir P, Allou N, Provenchère S, Berroeta C, Huisse M-G, Philip I, et al. Heparin-induced thrombocytopenia after cardiac surgery: an observational study of 1,722 patients. *J. Cardiothorac. Vasc. Anesth.* 2012;26(4):585-90.

[46] Pouplard C, Amiral J, Borg J-Y, Laporte-Simitsidis S, Delahousse B, Gruel Y. Decision analysis for use of platelet aggregation test, carbon 14-serotonin release assay, and heparin-platelet factor 4 enzyme-linked immunosorbent assay for diagnosis of heparin-induced thrombocytopenia. *Am. J. Clin. Pathol.* 1999;111(5):700-6.

[47] Warkentin T, Sheppard J, Moore J, Sigouin C, Kelton J. Quantitative interpretation of optical density measurements using PF4-dependent enzyme-immunoassays. *J. Thromb Haemost.* 2008;6(8):1304-12.

[48] Whitlatch NL, Kong DF, Metjian AD, Arepally GM, Ortel TL. Validation of the high-dose heparin confirmatory step for the diagnosis of heparin-induced thrombocytopenia. *Blood.* 2010;116(10):1761-6.

[49] Cuker A, Rux AH, Hinds JL, Cruz MD, Yarovoi SV, Brown IA, et al. Novel diagnostic assays for heparin-induced thrombocytopenia. *Blood.* 2013;121(18):3727-32.

[50] Sachais BS, Litvinov RI, Yarovoi SV, Rauova L, Hinds JL, Rux AH, et al. Dynamic antibody-binding properties in the pathogenesis of HIT. *Blood.* 2012;120(5):1137-42.

[51] Legnani C, Cini M, Pili C, Boggian O, Frascaro M, Palareti G. Evaluation of a new automated panel of assays for the detection of anti-PF4/heparin antibodies in patients suspected of having heparin-induced thrombocytopenia. *Thromb Haemost.* 2010;104(2):402.

[52] Davidson SJ, Ortel TL, Smith LJ. Performance of a new, rapid, automated immunoassay for the detection of anti-platelet factor 4/heparin complex antibodies. *Blood Coagul Fibrinolysis.* 2011;22(4):340-4.

[53] Selleng K, Schütt A, Selleng S, Warkentin TE, Greinacher A. Studies of the anti–platelet factor 4/heparin immune response: adapting the enzyme-linked immunosorbent

spot assay for detection of memory B cells against complex antigens. *Transfusion* (Paris). 2010;50(1):32-9.

[54] Sheridan D, Carter C, Kelton JG. A diagnostic test for heparin-induced thrombocytopenia. *Blood.* 1986;67(1):27-30.

[55] Greinacher A, Michels I, Kiefel V, Mueller-Eckhardt C. A rapid and sensitive test for diagnosing heparin-associated thrombocytopenia. *Thromb Haemost.* 1991;66(6):734-6.

[56] Prechel M, Walenga JM, editors. Heparin-induced thrombocytopenia: an update. *Semin Thromb Hemost;* 2012.

[57] Tomer A. A sensitive and specific functional flow cytometric assay for the diagnosis of heparin-induced thrombocytopenia. *Br. J. Haematol.* 1997;98(3):648-56.

[58] Vitale M, Tazzari P, Ricci F, Mazza MA, Zauli G, Martini G, et al. Comparison between different laboratory tests for the detection and prevention of heparin-induced thrombocytopenia. *Cytometry.* 2001;46(5):290-5.

[59] Mullier F, Bailly N, Cornet Y, Dubuc E, Robert S, Osselaer JC, et al. Contribution of platelet microparticles generation assay to the diagnosis of type II heparin-induced thrombocytopenia. *Thromb Haemost.* 2010 Jun;103(6):1277-81.

[60] Morel-Kopp M-C, Tan CW, Brighton TA, McRae S, Baker R, Tran H, et al. Validation of whole blood impedance aggregometry as a new diagnostic tool for HIT: results of a large Australian study. *Thromb Haemost.* 2012;107(3):575-83.

[61] Sachais BS, Rux AH, Cines DB, Yarovoi SV, Garner LI, Watson SP, et al. Rational design and characterization of platelet factor 4 antagonists for the study of heparin-induced thrombocytopenia. *Blood.* 2012;119(25):5955-62.

[62] Warkentin TE, Greinacher A, Koster A, Lincoff AM. Treatment and prevention of heparin-induced thrombocytopenia*: American college of chest physicians evidence-based clinical practice guidelines (8th edition). *CHEST Journal.* 2008;133(6_suppl):340S-80S.

[63] Warkentin TE, Elavathil LJ, Hayward CP, Johnston MA, Russett JI, Kelton JG. The pathogenesis of venous limb gangrene associated with heparin-induced thrombocytopenia. *Ann. Intern. Med.* 1997;127(9):804-12.

[64] Sheth S, DiCicco R, Hursting M, Montague T, Jorkasky D. Interpreting the International Normalized Ratio (INR) in individuals receiving argatroban and warfarin. *Thrombosis and Haemostasis-Stuttgart.* 2001;85(3):435-40.

[65] Hopkins CK, Goldfinger D. Platelet transfusions in heparin-induced thrombocytopenia: a report of four cases and review of the literature. *Transfusion* (Paris). 2008 Oct;48(10):2128-32.

[66] Refaai MA, Chuang C, Menegus M, Blumberg N, Francis CW. Outcomes after platelet transfusion in patients with heparin-induced thrombocytopenia. *J. Thromb Haemost.* 2010 Jun;8(6):1419-21.

[67] Pötzsch B, Klövekorn W-P, Madlener K. Use of heparin during cardiopulmonary bypass in patients with a history of heparin-induced thrombocytopenia. *N. Engl. J. Med.* 2000;343(7):515-.

[68] Wanaka K, Matsuo T, Matsuo M, Kaneko C, Miyashita K, Asada R, et al. Re-exposure to heparin in uremic patients requiring hemodialysis with heparin-induced thrombocytopenia. *J. Thromb Haemost.* 2010;8(3):616-8.

[69] Warkentin TE, Sheppard JA. Serological investigation of patients with a previous history of heparin-induced thrombocytopenia who are reexposed to heparin. *Blood.* 2014 Apr 17;123(16):2485-93.

[70] Selleng S, Haneya A, Hirt S, Selleng K, Schmid C, Greinacher A. Management of anticoagulation in patients with subacute heparin-induced thrombocytopenia scheduled for heart transplantation. *Blood.* 2008;112(10):4024-7.

[71] Paolucci F, Claviés M-C, Donat F, Necciari J. Fondaparinux Sodium Mechanism of Action. *Clin. Pharmacokinet.* 2002;41(2):11-8.

[72] Nagler M, Haslauer M, Wuillemin WA. Fondaparinux - data on efficacy and safety in special situations. *Thromb Res.* 2012 Apr;129(4):407-17.

[73] Schindewolf M, Steindl J, Beyer-Westendorf J, Schellong S, Dohmen PM, Brachmann J, et al. Frequent off-label use of fondaparinux in patients with suspected acute heparin-induced thrombocytopenia (HIT) - findings from the GerHIT multi-centre registry study. *Thromb Res. 2014* Mar 18.

[74] Baroletti S, Labreche M, Niles M, Fanikos J, Goldhaber SZ. Prescription of fondaparinux in hospitalised patients. *Thromb Haemost.* 2009;101(6):1091-4.

[75] Harenberg J, Jorg I, Fenyvesi T. Treatment of heparin-induced thrombocytopenia with fondaparinux. *Haematologica.* 2004;89(8):1017-8.

[76] Warkentin TE, Cook RJ, Marder VJ, Sheppard J-AI, Moore JC, Eriksson BI, et al. Anti–platelet factor 4/heparin antibodies in orthopedic surgery patients receiving antithrombotic prophylaxis with fondaparinux or enoxaparin. *Blood.* 2005;106(12):3791-6.

[77] Bhatt VR, Aryal MR, Shrestha R, Armitage JO. Fondaparinux-associated heparin-induced thrombocytopenia. *Eur. J. Haematol.* 2013 Jul 26;91(5):437-41.

[78] Warkentin TE. Fondaparinux: does it cause HIT? Can it treat HIT? *Expert Rev. Hematol.* 2010;3(5):567-81.

[79] Bhatt VR, Aryal MR, Armitage JO. Nonheparin anticoagulants for heparin-induced thrombocytopenia. *N. Engl. J. Med.* 2013 Jun 13;368(24):2333-4.

[80] Burch M, Cooper B. Fondaparinux-associated heparin-induced thrombocytopenia. *Proc. (Bayl Univ Med Cent).* 2012;25(1):13.

[81] Modi C, Satani D, Cervellione KL, Cervantes J, Gintautas J. Delayed-onset heparin-induced thrombocytopenia type-2 during fondiparinux (Arixtra) therapy. *Proc. West Pharmacol Soc.* 2009;52:5-7.

[82] Rota E, Bazzan M, Fantino G. Fondaparinux-related thrombocytopenia in a previous low-molecular-weight heparin (LMWH)-induced heparin-induced thrombocytopenia (HIT). *Thromb Haemost.* 2008 Apr;99(4):779-81.

[83] Salem M, Elrefai S, Shrit MA, Warkentin TE. Fondaparinux thromboprophylaxis-associated heparin-induced thrombocytopenia syndrome complicated by arterial thrombotic stroke. *Thromb Haemost.* 2010 Nov;104(5):1071-2.

[84] Warkentin TE, Chakraborty AK, Sheppard JA, Griffin DK. The serological profile of fondaparinux-associated heparin-induced thrombocytopenia syndrome. *Thromb Haemost.* 2012 Aug;108(2):394-6.

[85] Warkentin TE, Maurer BT, Aster RH. Heparin-induced thrombocytopenia associated with fondaparinux. *N. Engl. J. Med.* 2007 Jun 21;356(25):2653-5; discussion -5.

[86] Miranda AC, Donovan JL, Tran MT, Gore JM. A case of unsuccessful treatment of heparin-induced thrombocytopenia (HIT) with fondaparinux. *J. Thromb Thrombolysis.* 2012 Jan;33(1):133-5.
[87] Warkentin TE. HIT: treatment easier, prevention harder. *Blood.* 2012 Feb 2;119(5):1099-100.
[88] Warkentin TE. HIT paradigms and paradoxes. *J. Thromb Haemost.* 2011 Jul;9 Suppl 1:105-17.
[89] Annicchierico FJ, Alonso JL. Dabigatran for heparin-induced thrombocytopenia. *Mayo Clin Proc.* 2013 Sep;88(9):1036.
[90] Krauel K, Hackbarth C, Furll B, Greinacher A. Heparin-induced thrombocytopenia: in vitro studies on the interaction of dabigatran, rivaroxaban, and low-sulfated heparin, with platelet factor 4 and anti-PF4/heparin antibodies. *Blood.* 2012 Feb 2;119(5):1248-55.
[91] Mirdamadi A. Dabigatran, a direct thrombin inhibitor, can be a life-saving treatment in heparin-induced thrombocytopenia. *ARYA atherosclerosis.* 2013;9(1):112.
[92] Walenga JM, Prechel M, Hoppensteadt D, Escalante V, Chaudhry T, Jeske WP, et al. Apixaban as an alternate oral anticoagulant for the management of patients with heparin-induced thrombocytopenia. *Clin Appl Thromb Hemost.* 2013 Sep;19(5):482-7.
[93] Walenga JM, Prechel M, Jeske WP, Hoppensteadt D, Maddineni J, Iqbal O, et al. Rivaroxaban--an oral, direct Factor Xa inhibitor--has potential for the management of patients with heparin-induced thrombocytopenia. *Br. J. Haematol.* 2008 Oct;143(1):92-9.
[94] Schell AM, Petras M, Szczepiorkowski ZM, Ornstein DL. Refractory heparin induced thrombocytopenia with thrombosis (HITT) treated with therapeutic plasma exchange and rituximab as adjuvant therapy. *Transfus Apher Sci.* 2013 Oct;49(2):185-8.
[95] Abdel-Razeq HN, Bajouda AA, Khalil MM, Ashmeg AK. Treating heparin-induced thrombocytopenia. The unconventional way! *Saudi Med. J.* 2004;25(9):1258-60.
[96] Antonijevic NM, Savic NB, Perunicic J, Kovac M, Mikovic D, Stanojevic M, et al. Salvage late plasmapheresis in a patient with pulmonary embolism caused by heparin-induced thrombocytopenia primarily resistant to danaparoid sodium and lepirudin. *J. Clin. Apher.* 2006;21(4):252-5.
[97] Bouvier J, Lefevre P, Villain P, Elias A, Durand J, Juhan I, et al. Treatment of serious heparin-induced thrombocytopenia by plasma exchange: report on 4 cases. *Thromb Res.* 1989;51(3):335-6.
[98] Brady J, Riccio J, Yumen O, Makary A, Greenwood S. Plasmapheresis. A therapeutic option in the management of heparin-associated thrombocytopenia with thrombosis. *Am. J. Clin. Pathol.* 1991;96(3):394-7.
[99] Jaben EA, Torloni AS, Pruthi RK, Winters JL. Use of plasma exchange in patients with heparin-induced thrombocytopenia: A report of two cases and a review of the literature. *J. Clin. Apher.* 2011;26(4):219-24.
[100] Poullin P, Pietri PA, LefÈvre P. Heparin-induced thrombocytopenia with thrombosis: Successful treatment with plasma exchange. *Br. J. Haematol.* 1998;102(2):629-30.
[101] Welsby IJ, Um J, Milano CA, Ortel TL, Arepally G. Plasmapheresis and heparin reexposure as a management strategy for cardiac surgical patients with heparin-induced thrombocytopenia. *Anesth Analg.* 2010;110(1):30-5.

[102] Robinson JA, Lewis BE, editors. Plasmapheresis in the management of heparin-induced thrombocytopenia. *Semin Hematol*; 1999.
[103] Linkins L-A, Dans AL, Moores LK, Bona R, Davidson BL, Schulman S, et al. Treatment and Prevention of Heparin-Induced Thrombocytopenia: Antithrombotic Therapy and Prevention of Thrombosis: American College of Chest Physicians Evidence-Based Clinical Practice Guidelines. *CHEST Journal.* 2012;141 (2_suppl):e495S-e530S.
[104] Warkentin TE. Agents for the treatment of heparin-induced thrombocytopenia. *Hematol Oncol. Clin. North Am.* 2010 Aug;24(4):755-75, ix.
[105] Song X, Huhle G, Wang L, Hoffmann U, Harenberg J. Generation of anti-hirudin antibodies in heparin-induced thrombocytopenic patients treated with r-hirudin. *Circulation.* 1999;100(14):1528-32.
[106] Lobo B, Finch C, Howard A, Minhas S. Fondaparinux for the treatment of patients with acute heparin-induced thrombocytopenia. *Thromb Haemost.* 2008 Jan;99(1):208-14.
[107] Grouzi E, Kyriakou E, Panagou I, Spiliotopoulou I. Fondaparinux for the treatment of acute heparin-induced thrombocytopenia: a single-center experience. *Clin. Appl. Thromb Hemost.* 2010 Dec;16(6):663-7.
[108] Warkentin TE, Pai M, Sheppard JI, Schulman S, Spyropoulos AC, Eikelboom JW. Fondaparinux treatment of acute heparin-induced thrombocytopenia confirmed by the serotonin-release assay: a 30-month, 16-patient case series. *J. Thromb Haemost.* 2011 Dec;9(12):2389-96.
[109] Goldfarb MJ, Blostein MD. Fondaparinux in acute heparin-induced thrombocytopenia: a case series. *J. Thromb Haemost.* 2011 Dec;9(12):2501-3.
[110] Cegarra-Sanmartin V, Gonzalez-Rodriguez R, Paniagua-Iglesias P, Santamaria-Ortiz A, Cueva LF, Galan-Serrano J, et al. Fondaparinux as a Safe Alternative for Managing Heparin-Induced Thrombocytopenia in Postoperative Cardiac Surgery Patients. *J. Cardiothorac. Vasc. Anesth.* 2014 Jan 15.
[111] Benken ST, Tillman N, Dajani S, Shah A, Thomas T. A retrospective evaluation of fondaparinux for confirmed or suspected heparin-induced thrombocytopenia in left-ventricular-assist device patients. *J. Cardiothorac. Surg.* 2014;9:55.

In: Thrombocytopenia
Editor: Mckenzie G. Bell

ISBN: 978-1-63321-713-3

Chapter 7

Thrombocytopenia in Dengue, Its Complication and Treatments

***Somsri Wiwanitkit*[1] *and Viroj Wiwanitkit*[2]**
[1] Wiwanitkit House, Bangkhae, Bangkok Thailand
[2] Visiting Professor, Faculty of Medicine, University of Nis, Serbia

Abstract

Dengue is an important tropical infection caused by dengue mosquito vector. Annually, thousands cases of dengue can be seen in tropical zone. This infection classically manifests as an acute febrile illness with thrombocytopenia. Thrombocytopenia in dengue can be problematic and lead to fatality. Several complications of dengue thrombocytopenia can be seen in tropical medicine. In this brief article, the authors will review and discusses on the complication of dengue thrombocytopenia and its treatment.

Keywords: Dengue, thrombocytopenia, complication, treatment

Introduction

Dengue is an important tropical infection caused by dengue mosquito vector. The corresponding pathogenic virus is called dengue virus [1]. The disease is considered as one of the two most important mosquito - borne infectious disease (the other is malaria). This viral infection can be seen in many countries at present [1]. Annually, thousands cases of dengue can be seen in tropical zone. This infection classically manifests as an acute febrile illness with thrombocytopenia. The patient usually presents with a compliant of high fever that cannot be resolved by simple acetaminophen intake [1]. The clinical finding includes appearance of petichiae. This can be overt or simply trigger by applied of pressure by tourniquet test [2]. Also, in serious cases, bleeding can be important clinical features [3]. For laboratory investigation, the dengue triad as thrombocytopenia, atypical lymphocytosis and hemoconcentration are the hallmarks of infection [1]. Thrombocytopenia in dengue can be problematic and lead to fatality. Several complications of dengue thrombocytopenia can be seen in tropical medicine. In this brief article, the authors will review and discusses on the complication of dengue thrombocytopenia and its treatment.

Pathogenesis of Thrombocytopenia in Dengue

As noted, thrombocytopenia is an important clinical laboratory aberration in dengue. The important finding is the decreased number of platelet and alteration of other platelet parameters especially for mean platelet volume [4]. Lai et al. noted that "thrombocytopenia was very common and 84.6% patients had a platelet count less than 100,000/mm3 [5]." Another report in India showed that thrombocytopenia could be seen in about 61.39% of cases [6].

The interesting query is on the exact pathogenesis of thrombocytopenia in dengue. The interesting theory is on immunopathology. It is proposed that immune mimic might be an important underlying etiology of dengue. Wiwanitkit noted that "platelet CD61 might have an important role in causing hemorrhagic complication in dengue infection [7]." The functional similarity between dengue non structural protein 1 and platelet integrin/adhesin protein, CD61 is believed to be the explanation for the phenomenon [8]. Immunomimicking can result in cross destruction from virus to platelet and result in thrombocytopenia [7]. This phenomenon can be seen in acute phase of infection and corresponds to the finding of thrombocytopenia in a few days after onset of illness. And the spontaneous resolution of thrombocytopenia in dengue patient can be further explained by "weak binding affinity of immunoglobin G" comparing to immunoglobin M [9].

Complication of Dengue Thrombocytopenia

Thrombocytopenia is an important hematological problem. Since platelet is one of the three required components for blood coagulation (platelet, vascular and clotting factor), the abnormality of platelet can lead to hemorrhage. The well-known dengue hemorrhagic fever is the specific form of dengue that has the bleeding clinical feature. There are many complications of dengue thrombocytopenia. Bleeding in dengue can be seen at any sites. Some rare sites include gastrointestinal tract and genitourinary tract [3]. However, those bleeding complications are primary outcomes of dengue thrombocytopenia. There are also some rarely mentioned secondary complications due to dengue bleedings. Those important ones will be hereby presented and discussed.

1. Pituitary apoplexy

   Pituitary apoplexy can be secondary to thrombocytopenia due to dengue hemorrhagic fever [10]. Wildemberg et al. mentioned "dengue as a probable novel condition for pituitary apoplexy because it may be associated with multiple risk factors for pituitary infarction or bleeding [11]." Wildemberg et al. noted that pituitary apoplexy should be kept in mind in any dengue case with "a rapid onset of severe headache and vision defects, even in those without known pituitary adenomas [11]."

2. Subdural hematoma

An important bleeding site in dengue hemorrhagic fever is in neurological system. Adding to the bleeding, the secondary condition as hematoma can be seen. The problematic subdural hematoma can be observed and this can be fatal [12 - 13]. This condition of hemorrhagic encephalopathy usually occurs during convalescence and a successful recovery can be seen following surgery [14].

3. Acute respiratory failure

Acute respiratory failure is reported secondary to alveolar hemorrhage due to dengue thrombocytopenia [15].

4. Acute compartment syndrome

Acute compartment syndrome can be secondary to bleeding due to dengue thrombocytopenia [16 – 17].

Treatment for Dengue Thrombocytopenia

As noted, there are several clinical problems that can be complications of dengue thrombocytopenia. To manage dengue thrombocytopenia seems to be a very important therapeutic consideration in dengue management. As recommended, the most effective way for management of dengue in any form (hemorrhage/shock or not) is fluid replacement therapy with closed monitoring. There are also other treatment options but those options are usually not as effective as good fluid resuscitation.

1. Steroid therapy

Steroid therapy is considered useless. Shashidhara et al. concluded that "high dose dexamethasone regimen was not effective in achieving a higher rise in the platelet count in the acute stage of dengue fever [18]." Tam et al. noted that steroid therapy gave "no reduction in the development of shock or other recognized complications of dengue virus infection [19]."

2. Immunoglobulin therapy

Kharya et al. noted that "intravenous anti-D can possibly be a treatment option for refractory thrombocytopenia [20]" in dengue. Yadav et al. noted that immunoglobulin therapy could be dramatic improve the case with severe thrombocytopenia (<10,000/mm3) [21].

3. Platelet transfusion

Considering the pathogenesis as immunomimicking, platelet transfusion seems to be useless for correction of dengue thrombocytopenia. Khan Assir et al. reported that "platelet transfusion did not prevent development of severe bleeding or shorten time to cessation of bleeding and was associated with significant side effects [22]."

References

[1] Wiwanitkit V. Dengue fever *Expert Rev Anti Infect Ther.* 2010 Jul;8(7):841-5

[2] Wiwanitkit V. The tourniquet *Trop Doct.* 2005 Apr;35(2):127-8.

[3] Wiwanitkit V. Bleeding and other presentations in Thai patients with dengue *Clin Appl Thromb Hemost.* 2004 Oct;10(4):397-8.

[4] Wiwanitkit V. Mean platelet volume in the patients with dengue *Platelets.* 2004 May;15(3):185.

[5] Lai PC, Lee SS, Kao CH, Chen YS, Huang CK, Lin WR, Wann SR, Lin HH, Yen MY, Liu YC. Characteristics of a dengue *J Microbiol Immunol Infect.* 2004 Oct;37(5):266-70.

[6] Singh NP, Jhamb R, Agarwal SK, Gaiha M, Dewan R, Daga MK, Chakravarti A, Kumar S. The 2003 outbreak of Dengue fever in Delhi, India. *Southeast Asia* 2005 Sep;36(5):1174-8.

[7] Wiwanitkit V. Platelet CD61 might have an important role in causing hemorrhagic complication in dengue *Clin Appl Thromb Hemost.* 2005 Jan;11(1):112.

[8] Wiwanitkit V. A study on functional similarity between dengue *J Ayub Med Coll Abbottabad.* 2006 Jul-Sep;18(3):13-6.

[9] Wiwanitkit V. Weak binding affinity of immunoglobin G, an explanation for the immune mimicking theory in pathophysiologic findings in the recovery *Nanomedicine.* 2005 Sep;1(3):239-40.

[10] Tan SK, Seow CJ, Tan E, Chau YP, Dalan R. Pituitary Apoplexy Secondary to Thrombocytopenia Due to Dengue Hemorrhagic Fever: A Case Report and Review of Literature. *Endocr Pract.* 2013 Dec 10:1-19. [Epub ahead of print]

[11] Wildemberg LE, Neto LV, Niemeyer P, Gasparetto EL, Chimelli L, Gadelha MR. Association of dengue hemorrhagic fever with multiple risk factors for pituitary apoplexy. *Endocr Pract.* 2012 Sep-Oct;18(5):e97-e101.

[12] Mittal M, Jain N. Subdural haematoma and axonal polyneuropathy complicating dengue *BMJ Case Rep.* 2011 Jun 17;2011. pii: bcr1220103672.

[13] Jain N, Gutch M, Kumar V, Naik AK. A fatal combo of dengue *Neurol India.* 2012 Jan-Feb;60(1):105-6.

[14] Kumar R, Prakash O, Sharma BS. Dengue hemorrhagic fever: a rare presentation as atypical acute subdural hematoma. *Pediatr Neurosurg*. 2008;44(6):490-2.

[15] Cadélis G. Intra-alveolar hemorrhage associated with dengue and leptospirosis. *Rev Pneumol Clin.* 2012 Oct;68(5):323-6.

[16] Wiwanitkit S, Wiwanitkit V. Dengue hemorrhagic Fever and acute compartment syndrome *N Am J Med Sci.* 2013 Mar;5(3):245.

[17] Bandyopadhyay D, Mondal P, Samui S, Bishnu S, Manna S. Acute compartment syndrome *N Am J Med Sci.* 2012 Dec;4(12):667-8.

[18] Shashidhara KC, Murthy KA, Gowdappa HB, Bhograj A. Effect of high dose of steroid on plateletcount in acute stage of dengue *J Clin Diagn Res.* 2013 Jul;7(7):1397-400.

[19] Tam DT, Ngoc TV, Tien NT, Kieu NT, Thuy TT, Thanh LT, Tam CT, Truong NT, Dung NT, Qui PT, Hien TT, Farrar JJ, Simmons CP, Wolbers M, Wills BA. Effects of short-course oral corticosteroid therapy in early dengue infection in Vietnamese patients: a randomized, placebo-controlled trial. *Clin Infect Dis.* 2012 Nov;55(9):1216-24.

[20] Kharya G, Yadav SP, Katewa S, Sachdeva A. Management of severe refractory thrombocytopenia Pediatr Hematol Oncol. 2011 Nov;28(8):727-32.

[21] Yadav SP, Sachdeva A, Gupta D, Sharma SD, Kharya G. Control of massive bleeding in dengue hemorrhagic fever with severe thrombocytopenia by use of intravenous anti-D globulin. *Pediatr Blood Cancer.* 2008 Dec;51(6):812-3.
[22] Khan Assir MZ, Kamran U, Ahmad HI, Bashir S, Mansoor H, Anees SB, Akram J. Effectiveness of platelet transfusion *Transfus Med Hemother.* 2013 Oct;40(5):362-8.

Index

A

B

C

D

E

I

N

O

P

Q

R

U

V

W

Y